"*Flash Point* is a book for all of us. What author Christy Warren has captured is every human's struggle to feel safe, secure, attached, and connected. This is a life-saving book with the understanding that we must take care of ourselves along the way. Warren expertly outlines how she worked through many of her struggles and realistically writes to her failures along her journey even while trying to heal. Her journey is many of ours—her recovery can also be ours."

—Tom Satterly, retired CSM Delta Force
and author of *All Secure: A Special Operations Soldier's Fight
to Survive on the Battlefield and the Homefront*

"Christy Warren's powerful memoir of her struggle with PTSD is both heartbreaking and inspiring. It's a must-read for first responders and the clinicians who help them heal."

—Ellen Kirschman, PhD, public safety psychologist,
author of *I Love a Fire Fighter* and *I Love a Cop*,
and coauthor of *Counseling Cops*

"A tough and emotional read but a must-read. Christy dives deep into her life's journey of trauma and, more importantly, her healing and ultimate recovery. I cried and I laughed and I can honestly say this book has helped me dig into my never-ending healing process. If you need inspiration, Christy nails it."

—Clint Malarchuk, former NHL goaltender
and author of *A Matter of Inches*

"Christy captures the constant exposure to exigent calls a firefighter faces. Over time it takes a toll on our brains."

—Sig Wallen, firefighter for the San Francisco Fire Department

FLASH
POINT

FLASH POINT

A Firefighter's Journey Through PTSD

CHRISTY WARREN

SHE WRITES PRESS

Published 2023
Printed in the United States of America

Print ISBN: 978-1-64742-448-0
E-ISBN: 978-1-64742-449-7
Library of Congress Control Number: 2022918618

For information, address:
She Writes Press
1569 Solano Ave #546
Berkeley, CA 94707

Interior design by Katherine Lloyd, The DESK

She Writes Press is a division of SparkPoint Studio, LLC.

For all the rescuers who have
worn the blood and endured the screams
of those they serve.

AUTHOR'S NOTE

I first wish to note everything in this book is the telling of my story. I have no other motives, such as making anyone look bad. We all had and have our own struggles. Like watching nature shows, you feel compassion for the animal the story is following. If a mother tiger kills an antelope to feed her family, you are happy for the mother tiger. If the story follows an antelope herd and one gets devoured by a tiger, you will feel sad for the antelope. Everything in this book is true according to the memories my brain delivers when summoned.

There is debate as to how well and how far back we can remember. Everything I tell you is what lives inside my head. My family, coworkers, and anyone else may have a different version of what happened. I can only guarantee everything included in this book is as I remember it.

Also, most of the names have been changed to protect their privacy.

PROLOGUE

The heat of the afternoon intensified the smell of asphalt as I stepped out of the ambulance onto the two-lane highway. A sea of flashing red lights from several emergency vehicles encased the head-on accident. Firefighters scrambled, setting up equipment to tear open the car to remove the trapped occupants. Police officers asked questions and carefully made measurements, investigating the accident scene to determine what happened. A witness said the driver had drifted right, then overcorrected and crossed the centerline, just in front of a pickup truck traveling fifty-five miles per hour.

The two vehicles collided with enough force to tear her aorta. Her heart may have beat one more time after impact, but there wouldn't have been any blood to pump. The front end of her car was a mangled pile of crushed engine parts and the passenger compartment reduced to half its original size. The boy in the front seat, her four-year-old son, somehow alive, was the first one to be removed. There was barely room for me to crawl through the passenger side, over the center console, and into the back seat. My task was to handle her twelve-year-old son in the back seat. I had to keep him calm, while firefighters used hydraulic cutters, spreaders, and rams to rip and cut away the metal wreckage trapping him inside.

"Maaoom!" The boy screamed to his silent and still mother. There were no sentences or questions, just screaming.

His femur was broken completely through the skin, but his screams were only for his mother. The more he screamed and fought to get out, the more his femur separated. Amazed he could move his leg at all, I sat in the back seat perpendicular to him and struggled with him as he attempted to crawl through the center console. His royal blue shorts and white socks wicked at the blood.

His mother's head was tilted to the right at such an angle that her long brown hair lightly spread across my shoulder and my bare arm.

We finally peeled the car away from the boy. He continued to scream for his mom and thrash as we wrestled him onto the backboard and into the leg splint. He was put into an ambulance, while his mom was left behind in the front seat of her car.

The four-year-old ended up in the back of my ambulance. He was wrapped on a kid-size backboard with gauze around his head, his face flattened from hitting the dashboard. Only one of his eyes followed me as I maneuvered next to him.

"Where is my mom? Where is my mom?" he asked over and over, his jaw barely moving, as we sped to the hospital.

When we arrived, we handed off the little boy to the orchestrated chaos of the emergency room. He continued to ask for his mom. I didn't stay to listen to what they told him, if they told him anything. I just carried the EKG monitor and the oxygen tank back to my office on four wheels.

It would all be removed—the IV, EKG, and EKG patches; the gauze packaging, the plastic caps, and the gloves; the pieces of tape and suction tubing turned red. The blood would be cleaned from the floor of my ambulance where the boy had been. The blood on my uniform pants would come out in the wash.

But the silence from the front seat and the screams from the back seat would remain forever.

I was nineteen years old, an emergency medical technician, working for a private ambulance company. On any given day for the next twenty-five years of my career as a paramedic and a firefighter, whenever I smelled hot asphalt, my skin sensed that woman's hair on my arm and heard her boy's screams. No one ever taught me how to calm a twelve-year-old howling for his mother, who sat dead in the seat in front of him. No one prepared me to answer a four-year-old's questions about where his mom was, when she was so entangled in metal they had no other choice but to leave her body in the car as they towed it away. I convinced myself it was in his best interest to tell him my colleagues were helping her. Later I'd realize it was as much for him as it was for me.

The common expectation when a loved one goes to work or to the grocery store is that they'll come home. But sometimes they don't, and that's when I show up.

I was there, for example, after a father went to buy a gallon of milk and misjudged a turn, wrapping his car around a tree, ending his life. His son became fatherless and his wife a widow.

Day after day, I would run calls like this, listen to screams, and get my hands covered in blood and brains and vomit. After the response was complete and my job was done, I placed the wreckage in a box in my head and went to the next call or decided between tacos or a sandwich for lunch. Just like I'd done with the mother and her two little boys, I put each experience in the box, closed the lid, and continued my job.

Until one day the box got too full, the lid flew open, and the insides blew all over everything.

PART I

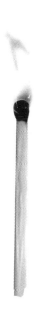

CHAPTER ONE

On the day Mom and I made the two-hour drive from Menlo Park to UC Davis for move-in day at the dorms, the warmth of the afternoon heightened the substantial smell of the nearby pig barn. We quickly found the three-story dorm made of white concrete that would be my home for the next ten months. Parents and new students milled throughout the hallways. Everyone wore cheerful smiles peppered with apprehension. Mom wore a T-shirt that said, "It's not pretty being easy" on the front.

We walked up the stairs to the third floor and found my room. The door was open and inside a young woman was arranging her belongings.

"Are you Cheryl?" I asked.

When she turned around, she flashed one of the biggest smiles I had ever seen—one that spread across her entire face—and she reached out to shake my hand.

"Hi! Yes, I'm Cheryl!" Her smile stayed on her face. "Do you need any help?" she asked.

In that moment, I knew Cheryl and I were going to get along great. She just oozed positivity and kindness without an ounce of judgment.

"I think I got it, but thank you."

Other dorm residents filed their way in and out of our room, introducing themselves. As more people entered the room, Cheryl asked me, "Do you have any dental floss? I have something stuck in my teeth, and I can't find mine anywhere."

Before I had a chance to react, Mom jumped in.

"Oh my! Running out of dental floss is like running out of cigarettes! I'm sure I have some in my purse."

The handful of people milling around stopped what they were doing and laughed. Mom beamed; she loved an audience. She always seemed to be looking for the moment she could say the thing that would evoke a laugh, drawing everyone's focus to her. It drove me crazy, so I did what I did best—tuned her out. I stood back and leaned against the wall, while she continued to work the room.

As usual, she was the star, and I was invisible.

Our three-story dorm housed what became one big family. Rarely did anyone lock their doors. And best of all, I was loved and accepted.

In school prior to college, I'd rarely fit in. I was a tomboy, so while the other girls were in ballet and Girl Scouts, I played baseball and refused to wear a skirt. In first grade, I'd regularly get thrown into a large swath of juniper bushes by schoolyard bullies. In junior high, the popular kids relished making fun of me for the clothes I wore. I had the mouth of a sailor and took basketball in PE way too seriously. I was truly always picked last, and few people acknowledged I existed. For most of my life, I'd felt like a square peg trying to fit in a round hole.

The summers were different. Every summer from the age of nine, with my green army duffle bag, I'd climb on a big yellow bus with all the other campers and head to the Caritas Creek Summer Camp in Mendocino. The counselors and staff sang camp songs and danced with excitement as the bus pulled up. I got more love and hugs during that ten-day session than I did all year long at home. I mattered there.

At the end of the session, I'd take the same yellow bus home. Before I even stepped off the bus, a plan formulated in my head on how I could go back in a few days for the next session. My mom and the camp director always found a way.

When I became a counselor at thirteen, I discovered the joy of working with kids, and I stayed in that role until I was eighteen. Caritas Creek focused on fostering community and was a safe place to experience unconditional love. They delivered a message to us kids that we mattered for exactly who we were. We were taught to love and respect one another regardless of our skin color, socioeconomic status, family dynamics, and anything else that might set someone apart or cause them to stand out as different.

At summer camp, I found structure, accountability, and safety. When I became a camp counselor, I realized if I became a teacher, I could teach other kids the same things so meaningful to me—they were valued and enough, just the way they were.

While this was my frame of mind when I arrived at UC Davis with my declared major in human development, I was more interested in partying and spending time with my new friends than studying. Luckily, I wrote well, so even though I usually started my papers hours before they were due, I maintained decent grades.

Only once did I try to start a paper several days before it was due. I sat in front of my computer with the word "Tittle" on the screen. (Always a good start when the only word on the page is misspelled.) It was all I could come up with for days. It seemed I was only capable of getting shit done if it was the very last minute.

For two quarters, I partied Thursdays, Fridays, and Saturdays.

I slept until noon on Mondays. Sometimes I'd go to class, most often I'd sleep. I'd start papers right before they were due. Repeat.

Then, one evening toward the middle of spring quarter, one of my dormmates popped his head in our room and said, "It's Thursday night. Grab your cash and any beer you can find and meet in the common room."

About fifteen of us pooled our money and ordered pizza. While we shoved slices in our faces, the conversation shifted to what we wanted to be when we grew up. After a couple of my peers talked about their own dreams, I spoke up.

"I wish I could be a doctor," I said.

A quiet fell over the room.

A friend said, "Then why don't you be one?"

My brain froze for a few seconds before I formulated a sentence. "It never crossed my mind that I could be a doctor. But hell, why not be a doctor?"

I'd always thought only fancy, smart people became doctors. I never entertained the idea I could be good enough or smart enough to be a part of this group.

When sophomore year rolled around, I started on my career path to become a doctor. Immediately, I changed my major to physiology and I signed up for classes required for medical school. Cheryl and four of our friends from the dorms moved into a condominium together. The vibe of living off-campus was mellower, and I studied more. I still enjoyed my weekends, but not in the same intense and constant way I had freshman year. I also knew I had to get top grades to get into medical school.

I had always loved blood, guts, skeleton parts, the brain, and the heart. But the first year of a physiology major didn't delve into any of that. Instead, I took chemistry, calculus, microbiology, and other grueling, dry science and math courses. The labs were dull and frustrating. I needed something more than trying to get my Bunsen burner tuned just right and counting drops of water distilled out of some blue liquid.

Since I was first-semester sophomore year and premed, I joined a student group of aspiring doctors. One of the activities of the group was to shadow doctors at a hospital. We had to buy and wear white doctor coats and name tags. I couldn't wait to put on my doctor coat and walk around the hospital like I was someone. People would look at me and think, *There goes a doctor!* And more important, now, finally, I would get to see a severed arm.

On the first day of rounds at the hospital, our director of the program met us in the hospital lobby. We stood in a circle, while he reminded us anything short of complete professionalism would not be tolerated. The speech was clearly meant to intimidate this group of nineteen- and twenty-year-olds into behaving like adults.

I walked through the sterile and empty hallways to locate the two doctors I was assigned to shadow. I introduced myself and shook their hands. We all wore the same white coat. They first took me to the cafeteria, where we spent the next hour sitting around a pink Formica table discussing one of their patient's lab results.

"It looks like we are going to have to tap his belly again," Doctor #1 finally said.

I envisioned a beer tap and imagined the doctors jamming a big, long, sharp needle into the patient and withdrawing a yellowish fluid. We got up from the table and headed to the patient's room.

"How are you feeling today?" Doctor #1 asked the patient.

The patient struggled to get the words out. "Not so good."

Doctor #2 gently tapped in several areas on the patient's

grossly distended belly. He said, "Yeah, we are going to have to tap your belly again. Sorry about that."

We went to the nurses' station, where Doctor #2 wrote in the patient's chart. I slouched in a chair and swiveled back and forth, counting faded linoleum squares on the floor. There was not one severed arm in sight. I didn't even get to watch the belly tap. My time at the hospital looking like a doctor was not exciting. Sitting in a hospital cafeteria and reading lab results was not my idea of a good time. I questioned whether this doctor thing was the right choice for me.

Maybe if I had spent some time in the emergency room, I'd have continued my studies to be a doctor. But fate had other plans.

One day, filling up time before my next class, I started reading one of the cork bulletin boards that garnished every building on campus. There was my summons on half a sheet of bright yellow paper—a flyer for an emergency medical technician (EMT) class being taught on campus, four hours every Wednesday night.

EMT class? After watching the TV show *Emergency!*, about two Los Angeles firefighters/paramedics, for years when I was a kid, the words on this yellow piece of paper lit a fire under me. Maybe this was where I'd finally see some severed body parts. I couldn't sign up fast enough.

While I bided my time waiting for my EMT class to start, I became even more obsessed with that world and what waited for me. A fire engine or an ambulance would drive by, and I'd stare intently, hoping to catch a glimpse of the inside. I wanted to know where they were going and what happened. This EMT class, I knew, was going to be what I had been searching for.

With my new EMT textbook in hand, I pedaled my hand-me-down, Wizard-of-Oz, Dorothy bike back to my condo as fast as my legs would take me. Unlike my chemistry book, which I tossed aside and didn't open unless I had to, the EMT book was engrossing and all-consuming. I flipped through the pages and focused on the pictures of broken limbs, serious car accidents, gunshot wounds, and EMT equipment. I took the book with me wherever I went, even into the bathroom. I scoured every line before my first class even started.

I couldn't have articulated what was so attractive about the subject matter. What was it that sucked me in like a tractor beam to these pictures and the potential of taking care of someone with a gunshot wound or an arm cut off?

I now realize the answer. Whether it is an accident scene or a fire truck driving by, everyone looks. Drivers on the freeway slow down and rubberneck, desperately trying to get a glimpse of what happened.

I would be where everyone looked. With the knowledge from the book and an EMT certification, I would be in the middle of the action. People would watch to see what I was doing and maybe even think of me as a hero. As long as I had the uniform on, I would never be invisible.

CHAPTER TWO

My entire childhood was chaos. At four years old, I stood between my fiercely arguing parents and held out my arms, as if trying to split up two boxers in the ring, begging them to stop.

"I'm leaving for good!" My dad screamed before slamming the door and driving off.

Shortly after, my parents divorced. They were so young, just kids themselves when they got married at nineteen and twenty-one. There's a picture of my mom on their wedding day in 1969, wearing her wedding dress, three months pregnant with me. She held a glass of champagne and smoked a cigarette.

After they divorced, I no longer had a house I called my home. I floated between other people's homes—my mom's house and my dad's house. There was no longer "my house." Kodi, my younger brother of three years, was my one consistent family member. Every other Friday night, Mom would take us from her house and drop us off at the train station. When we were only ten and seven, we took the train together from Menlo Park to Daly City to go to our dad's house. At least we were together.

About a year after the divorce, Mom remarried and my brother and I moved in with her creepy new husband and his older son. My new stepdad introduced us to drugs, alcohol, and nudity.

He often walked around the house in nothing but a brown ter-rycloth bathrobe that hung open. One night, I walked into the living room to find him sitting by the fireplace completely naked. The house always smelled of musk and weed. The carpet was so flea-infested that when I walked around with white socks on, they would quickly be covered in black dots.

I desperately wanted my mom's attention, but she seemed mostly indifferent to me—an apathy that worsened after my parents' divorce.

Some time after we moved in with the creepy new husband, determined to somehow grab my mom's attention, I headed for the tree fort at the end of our street, planning to jump off. As I slowly climbed the two-by-fours nailed into the huge oak tree, I daydreamed about being injured and my mom tending to me with love and care. I climbed onto the plywood platform and sat with my legs dangling over the end, scouring my heart for cour-age. I wondered if it would work. I hoped I'd be seriously injured or even die. *Maybe then she'd pay attention to me.*

I stood up, looked down at the ground, which seemed so far away, and jumped.

I landed on my feet with a *thwack*! I fell forward into the dirt and lay there, face down with my eyes closed, sensing pain but only in my feet.

After a long moment, I opened my eyes and sat up. All of me was intact. I couldn't find any injuries. I stood up and brushed off my pants and shirt. Disappointed and embarrassed, I hoped no one saw me.

I was nine when Mom divorced her creepy husband and we moved again, this time into a cleaner house, maybe due to the hardwood floors. Mom was always quick to get a new boyfriend, and when she did, she'd completely disappear. When she was home, she talked about how wonderful her new guy was and all the great things they did together. Meanwhile, I wore the same hoodie every day to cover up the old clothes I was embarrassed to be seen in.

Mom talked about one wealthy boyfriend in particular. She went away on trips with him, and when she returned, she'd tell me about the fabulous time they'd had together. On one trip, the wealthy guy's son went with them. When I came back from my dad's one weekend, she couldn't wait to share her "good news."

"Oh Christy," she said, "his son is such a wonderful kid. I can't even explain to you what a wonderful time we all had together."

I stood in disbelief. How could she not know this made me think she'd rather be with someone else besides me? I must be the problem. I must not be worth spending time with.

At times she'd spend the night at her boyfriend's house and leave me at home alone. A tangled ball of fear and heartbreak would start in my throat and land hard in the pit of my stomach as I watched her walk out the door. I'd plead with her to stay. I was only twelve.

Drugs followed my mom to this house. She and her friends smoked a lot of weed. People came over with large boxes of pot and a scale. They sat at our dining room table, separating the buds and the seeds. The leaves and the buds were weighed and put into little baggies. My mom and her friends worked around the table, chatting as if they were making tamales. This became a regular occurrence.

Eventually, the white powder showed up. Mom and her friends snorted lines with a cut-down drinking straw and one-dollar bills. Parties came with the drugs, and Mom sure could throw a party. My house often rumbled with loud music and the voices of drunk, high strangers.

Outside of the house, my mom often drove drunk. One night, we were coming back from a wedding on the coast. The roads wound up and down a mountainside.

As we descended, Mom exclaimed, laughing, "Let's see if we can make it in the dark!" and she turned the headlights off.

I kept my eyes straight ahead and braced for when the car left the cliff.

We somehow managed to make the sweeping curve to the left. Mom let out a scream of joy and flipped the lights back on. I said nothing. I was more annoyed than afraid. I knew fear wouldn't do me any good. I'd learned to turn my emotions off a long time ago.

It would be many years before I learned that growing up in chaos primed me to function well in chaos.

Kodi was nine and I was twelve when he decided to live full time with my dad and stepmom. We still spent weekends together, but on Sunday nights we split up to separate homes. My one consistent family member became another weekend family member.

After Kodi moved, my mom spent a lot of time crying on the couch. She loved to write and filled yellow legal pad after yellow legal pad. One day, I found one of these pads in her room and read about the devastation imposed upon her when my brother chose to live with his father. In disbelief, I sat on the floor with her pad in my lap.

How can she not give a shit about us and then suddenly be this upset because Kodi left? She ignores me and yet she's this worked up over Kodi moving out? If I move out, will she even care? Will she even notice?

⌒

I found safety at my dad's house, since life was more normal there. We had plenty of food, and my dad and stepmom prepared meals for Kodi and me. We ate dinner at the table together, we brushed our teeth, and we'd be tucked into bed. They never left us home alone. There were no drugs, no drinking, and appropriate boundaries were always in place.

But there was a cost. He'd tell me what a burden I was to him and often told me I ruined his weekend because he had to drive in traffic to pick me up, take me home, or take me to my soccer or baseball games. He had a wild temper and at times, it would get the best of him. He'd come at me, his face red-hot with anger, fist clenched, and growling. "You snotty little shit!"

I wondered if he'd finally follow through and hit us. He always seemed to be mad at us for something—even Jason, the son he'd had with my stepmom, who was ten years younger than me.

I always felt responsible for both of my brothers. I needed to provide the love and acceptance they weren't getting and make sure they knew they were loved. This expectation of responsibility for both would extend into adulthood.

CHAPTER THREE

After completing my Wednesday night classroom portion, I
had to complete twenty-four hours of ride-alongs. I arrived
at the ambulance station as excited and nervous as a new kid on
the first day of school. I stopped at the front door of the station
and took a deep breath. Would I be cool enough so the paramedics and EMTs would like me? I couldn't wait to see these heroes
in action.

I knocked, and someone inside yelled, "It's open!"

I gave myself the once-over, making sure everything was in
place. My required dark pants, white shirt, and EMT student
name tag all seemed in order. I pushed the door open to a living
room with ratty old couches and a blaring TV. A few paramedics
and EMTs sat around watching whatever was on and shoveling
food in their faces. The rest were emerging from the kitchen,
plates in hand, their boots noisy on the well-worn linoleum floor.

Five men and one woman wore white, uniform, button-up
shirts with official patches and dark-blue pants. They piled their
plates high with lasagna, salad, and garlic bread. They ate with
purpose. One of them said something to me, but I couldn't
understand him through his mouthful of food. I stood in awe
while the rest of them ignored me.

They still shoveled in hot marinara sauce, cheese, and noodles when the bells went off, dispatching them to a call.

After shoveling several more bites of food into his mouth, one guy said to me, "Come with us. Let's go see what bullshit they're calling us for."

I followed the crew outside and climbed into the back of the ambulance—and in doing so, I stepped into a whole new world.

The six-minute drive to the scene seemed more like two minutes. I opened the back doors and climbed down the steps with my gloves on, ready to help save a life.

Once out of the ambulance, I looked around for the blood and guts. I only found several cops milling around a guy who wore a pair of jeans and handcuffs, as he stood in the headlights of a police car. The guy was high as a kite. Even though nothing was happening, everything moved fast. From hearing the cops and paramedics talk, I figured out the guy had to go to the hospital to be medically cleared so the cops could take him to jail. We all climbed back into the ambulance.

I smelled something horrible coming from my shoes. I lifted my foot up to find human poop all over the bottom of my shoe. Stepping in poop was disgusting, but somehow it made me feel more like "one of the guys."

For eight hours, I sat in the back of the ambulance, listened to the siren, watched our flashing red lights reflect off of buildings and other cars, and witnessed what it meant to be an EMT. This was much more fun than sitting in the cafeteria discussing bilirubin and alanine aminotransferase levels. I was hooked.

Immediately after getting my EMT card in late spring of my sophomore year, I attached it to the back of the sun visor in my car. I imagined myself happening upon an accident, proudly announcing to everyone I was an EMT, and then saving them all.

As the UC Davis school year came to an end, I never had the occasion to roll up on an accident or save everyone on site. But in class one day, I did happen to glimpse a Help Wanted ad for EMTs for Solano Ambulance in a loose newspaper.

I'd been searching for something to do that summer. *What the hell, I'll apply.*

As soon as I got home, I dialed the phone number in the ad. The lady on the phone said to come in, fill out an application, and my interview would happen at the same time.

Solano Ambulance was housed in an old, tan, two-story building with dark-brown trim. It had once been a firehouse. I walked through the front door into a cloud of cigarette smoke. To the right of the lobby, just on the other side of a Dutch door with the top open, sat the ambulance dispatcher. She talked into a microphone while punching a clock with yellow manila cards.

I walked into the office area on the left, where the receptionist introduced herself and handed me an application. When I completed the form, she sent me up the brown, carpeted stairs to the operations manager's office for the interview.

I walked in to find a super-tall guy seated at his desk. He rose, introduced himself as Tom Lee, and shook my hand.

"Have a seat," he said. "Leave the door open."

As he reviewed my application, a paramedic walked in and complained about a shift he was scheduled to work. The operations manager told him he had to work that day. After he left, another guy walked in and asked for some paperwork to be signed.

While signing the paperwork, Tom asked me, "Do you play basketball?"

I had no idea why he asked the question, but I nodded. "Yeah, I played in high school."

He gave me an approving look, and we talked about basketball for the next twenty minutes.

Eventually, he asked, "When can you start?"

"As soon as school ends, in about a week."

"We can hire you," he said. "You just have to pass the physical agility test."

Grateful for the weightlifting class I took, which had bulked up my skinny arms a tad, I nodded and smiled.

I showed up the following week for the test. They had me carry a bunch of bags full of equipment up and down the stairs. I carried a gurney with a person on it up and down those stairs. The gurneys we used back then were two-man gurneys. There had to be a person on each end of the gurney to lower it down almost to the ground, which folded up the gurney legs underneath. Then each person moved to a side of the gurney, and they picked up the whole thing and loaded it into the ambulance. This twisted our loaded backs in a way they were never meant to be twisted—but I was young and strong, and I managed fine.

I passed the test with no mistakes. I was going to be an actual EMT and work on an ambulance. Now when I watched the reflection of the red lights out the window, it would be me rushing to save someone.

CHAPTER FOUR

I bought my uniforms and had the official patches sewn on them. I was so excited to wear dark-blue, polyester, gas-station pants. I wore them all day like a superhero's cape. I became someone important, someone who mattered. I was nineteen years old and headed toward everything I'd ever wanted.

After a couple days of orientation, I had my first shift in the city of Benicia. It was a twenty-four-hour shift on a BLS (basic life support unit).

A BLS unit is an ambulance with two EMTs on it, while an ALS (advanced life support) unit is an ambulance with one EMT and one paramedic. They look the same except for the words "Paramedic Unit" emblazoned across the side.

My partner, Griff, was built like a linebacker and had a lot of hair, including a hearty mustache, but he was gentle as a bunny.

The first day dragged like it had a piano tied around it. I sat on the brown, overstuffed couch and stared at the red dispatch phone willing it to ring. Finally, around 3:00 p.m., the phone rang. My first 911 call. I ran out the door like I'd been shot out of a cannon.

I was new, so Griff drove us to our first call—a motor vehicle accident on the freeway. The car accident had been minor and the call straightforward. Still, the excitement of being there sent tingles all over my body. We took the patient to the hospital and headed back to our station.

The phone didn't ring again until about 8:00 p.m. This time the call was for a woman with abdominal pain.

I sprinted the entire twenty feet to the ambulance. This would be my first time driving to a call, and this call was code three, which meant using lights and sirens. I jumped into the driver's seat and slammed the door shut. I flipped on the lights and siren and punched the accelerator to the floor, not letting up except to make turns. A manic laugh belted out of me as I blasted through the first stop sign. I then blew through all the stop signs and every red light.

Griff had one hand on the roof and one hand on the dash, bracing himself, and he screamed at me the entire way. I was so high on adrenaline, I only heard the wail of the siren and not anything Griff said.

When we arrived on scene and I threw the ambulance into park, I looked over at Griff and all the color had drained from his face. I couldn't figure out why he wasn't feeling the same high I was.

With a red face and bulging eyes he choked out, "Almost killed me . . . That's not how we drive code three . . . Holy fuck . . . " were among some of the choice phrases he used.

All the way back from the hospital, Griff gave me a spirited lesson on driving code three, randomly punctuated by "holy fuck."

We worked a Kelly schedule, which meant I had rotating twenty-four-hour shifts. I would work Monday, Wednesday, and Friday and then get four days off, and it continued rotating. There were so many extra shifts needing to be filled that I worked much more than the regular schedule.

For my third shift on Friday of my brand-new career, I worked a twenty-four-hour shift in Vallejo. We spent the first part of the day transporting people from convalescent homes . . . so many of them trapped in their useless bodies. Their hearts continued to pump, but these people had no life. Even at my young age, I realized I never wanted to be in a place like this. I treated these people with compassion and empathy but mostly tried not to look. Running these calls was not what I wanted to be doing, but it was enough for now since I, insignificant me, worked on an ambulance. I walked through the emergency room like I belonged there because I did.

When I was first drawn to be an EMT, I never thought about how the job would bring me into the homes of so many people. I'd walk into lives filled with child neglect and parental anger, many of those scenes familiar to me.

One Christmas Eve around 2:00 a.m., our call brought us to a patient who had fallen in the bathroom and struck her head. Her breath reeked of alcohol and a male adult in the apartment was outrageously high. The woman had a serious head injury, but my focus was continually pulled back to the toddler walking around wearing only a diaper. I saw his neglect and felt his loneliness. *What in the fuck is wrong with people?* I wanted to scoop the kid up and take care of him. But I couldn't because I had to take care of his mother, who fell from being drunk.

However, I saw another side of parenthood on those calls. On a different night, my partner and I brought a patient to the emergency room. A hanging curtain separated the room. As we transferred our patient to the hospital bed, we heard a woman talking to a doctor on the other side of the curtain, telling him she thought her young daughter had an ear infection.

What the hell? I thought. *My mom never took me to the ER in the middle of the night.*

I remembered waking up in the middle of the pitch-black night a few times with my ear feeling like a burning knife had been stuck in it. I must have been seven when one night I laid in bed, finding the courage to wake my mom up, hoping this time she would help me. I knew I shouldn't bother her—whenever I had nightmares, she always told me to go back to bed and not wake her up—but this time the pain was unbearable. I shoved the covers back and walked to my mom's room. I crept up to her side of the bed and gently patted her arm.

"Mom. Hey, Mom."

She woke up. "What's the matter?"

"My ear hurts really, really bad."

"Go back to bed and don't wake me up again. I'll deal with it in the morning."

I turned around and went back to my room. I crawled into bed and the pain kept me awake the rest of the night.

That night in the emergency room, as I rolled the gurney out of our patient's room, I tilted my head toward the curtain to listen. It had never occurred to me that parents took their children to the hospital in the middle of the night when they were in pain. Throughout my career, middle-of-the-night ER visits by parents and their kids with ear infections was a regularity. Each time, a sense of comfort filled me to know another child wouldn't have to endure a night of pain and loneliness . . . that a child was being taken care of and one less person weighed on my shoulders to help. I was supposed to fix and save everyone whose life intersected with mine.

After working on the BLS ambulance for three months, I wanted more. There was rarely anything to be done or fix or to challenge me. I'd offer a hand to hold or compassion to make someone extra comfortable during the ambulance ride, but none of those small gestures fulfilled the impact I wanted to have. So when a spot opened up on an ALS unit, I seized it. Now I'd work with a paramedic and we'd answer 911 calls instead of what I came to see as just giving patients a ride home from the hospital.

My second shift on the ALS unit was a response to a call in the afternoon on Highway 680 in Benicia. A car with five people inside rolled off the freeway and up a short embankment. Several emergency vehicles with flashing red lights lined the shoulder of the freeway. We pulled over and parked in front of the line and scampered through twenty feet of tall, dry grass. There were two clumps of firefighters bending over each patient who'd been ejected. A couple of California Highway Patrol officers studied the damaged asphalt and the divots left in the ground from the car.

As I approached, everything in my head went quiet. The noise muffled as if I were underwater. A silver four-door sedan lay right side up, facing the wrong way on top of a level embankment. The body of the front-seat passenger, still inside the vehicle, slumped against his door. Something hung out the window opening. As I got closer, I could see the passenger's head had been compressed and flattened as if in a cartoon. He was obviously dead. Time slowed to a crawl as I stood and stared for a few long moments.

My paramedic partner calling for supplies pulled me from my trance. The sound came back on in my head as if I surfaced from a deep dive. In an instant, this family was torn to pieces. One was dead, two others had been ejected from the car while it rolled, and two others, the ones wearing their seat belts, had walked away without a scratch.

I worked quickly on one of the seriously injured patients who had been ejected. As we carried him strapped to a backboard, I looked back at the car on the side of the road. Quiet fell again. The two who had walked away frantically talked on their cell phones, pacing back and forth in the tall dry grass, desperate to get ahold of the rest of the family still driving north, headed to Sacramento to watch an airshow. The firefighters, cops, and the other paramedics moved like a fast-paced choreographed dance, except for the mangled teenager in the front seat, so quiet and still.

The people in the car were just a nice family out to spend a day together. These people looked forward to spending the day with the people they loved. In only an instant, their lives would never be the same. I stuffed the dead teenager and the distraught family into the box in my head and closed the lid.

After working as an EMT that summer, I continued working full-time and attended school at UC Davis part-time. I took two classes fall quarter 1990 and failed them both. I had no interest in studying, nor did I have the time or energy to do so. I only wanted to be on the ambulance. The more chaotic the call, the more serenity settled over me.

Since I worked twenty-four-hour shifts, I had a work bag, which I never unpacked. I'd remove my dirty clothes, wash them, then put them back. It was something I was used to. I'd had the same "always-packed" bag throughout my childhood, too. Every other weekend when I traveled to my dad's, I'd bring a bag of clothes and belongings. No wonder it was so easy for me to slide into this job.

As I settled into my new role as an ALS EMT, my dad moved from Half Moon Bay to Oregon. Kodi was still in high school, and Mom agreed to move from Menlo Park to Half Moon Bay so he didn't have to change high schools.

From what I saw, Mom took decent care of Kodi. I resented it because she'd hardly looked after me when I lived with her.

Between my dad regularly getting over-the-top furious with his kids and my mom not being interested in her daughter, I kept thinking, *There must be something wrong with me. If I wasn't defective, they would love and care about me.*

This belief of not being enough still lived somewhere inside my job. If I was speeding to save a life, there couldn't be anything inherently wrong with me. After the initial excitement of doing this for several months wore off, I felt inadequate being "just" an EMT. I wanted to be a paramedic. The cool kids were paramedics. I avoided answering questions regarding the difference between an EMT and a paramedic. And then I'd hesitate when I had to tell them I was only an EMT.

"You will never think you are enough," a close friend warned me. "When you become a paramedic, you will say, 'I am just a paramedic, not a firefighter-paramedic,' and on and on."

Still, I couldn't help thinking, *Maybe if I am a paramedic, I will actually become someone.*

I blew off what my friend said, but I kept the thought somewhere in my brain. I would never be enough. My entire life was always about the destination and never the journey. I believed I had to be the best or I was nothing. To never be enough, to never have been enough, entered me in a race where I'd do everything in my power to win. I did not see or hear anything except the finish line, which moved farther away right when I thought I was about to cross it.

This was my existence, and it was exhausting. If I could just reach the finish line, I'd be okay. I'd finally be enough.

But when the finish line is always moving, the impossibility of reaching it wears on you. Not reaching it means invisibility; it means worthlessness. And it's an impossible measure to reach and so you're destined to fail.

For a year I worked my ass off at *just* being an EMT. Then, in September 1991, I applied and was accepted into UCSF's paramedic school.

I dropped out of Davis for the winter and spring quarters with the idea I'd go back in the fall. Putting myself through the nine-month program full time became my singular focus. Picking up my paramedic textbook was almost as exciting as when I first got my EMT book. This book had even more pictures but also significantly more text.

The first part of paramedic school, the didactic, was all classroom. The next part was clinical—eight hours in the operating room, where I learned to intubate real, live humans. And the last part was the internship. I would spend 480 hours on an ambulance and work alongside a paramedic as the extra on the ambulance.

I arrived at 7:30 a.m. at the station for the first morning of my internship, proudly wearing my "Paramedic Intern" badge. I only had to wait fifteen minutes for a call to come in. It was for a cardiac arrest at a convalescent home.

I was thrilled; many interns wait and wait to get a code, while my first call was code. I had no idea at the time that call would set the tone for the rest of my career.

Codes are important in an internship; they give you the opportunity to learn medical and leadership skills, and to practice handling a great deal of stress getting a person's heart beating again in only a little time. Yet, I found codes easy because there was no sorting out what was wrong; they were not breathing, and their heart had stopped. I had to get the heart pumping and the lungs breathing again. I also knew once someone had gone into cardiac arrest, the chances of survival were very slim.

When we arrived at the con home, I jumped out of the ambulance with the medical bags in my hands. We stepped inside and walked through the front room and hallways, both filled with old men and women slowly roaming about in their wheelchairs. They had no awareness of what was going on. We walked into the patient's room with our medical bags. An elderly woman lying in bed watched us walk past her bed to her roommate's bed. A flimsy curtain was pulled closed between the two of them, as if it provided some privacy. We lifted her out of her bed and gently placed her on the floor to do CPR. I began giving directions to my partners and the fire department crew while I intubated her and started an IV, giving her all the proper medications.

Not more than ten minutes had passed before we loaded her onto the gurney and wheeled her to the ambulance. The woman was pronounced dead shortly after we arrived at the emergency room. Even though we didn't save her, I was proud of the job I'd done. And I was glad she wasn't suffering anymore.

Shortly after that first code, my unit was dispatched to another critical call. A six-year-old boy had ridden his skateboard down his driveway. His wheel hit a small rock, stopping his skateboard but not him. He landed in the road just as a car was driving by. His head got caught under the car and he was dragged about twenty feet until his ear was scraped off and the white of his skull exposed.

The fire department arrived on the scene just before us and had already lifted the car up and off of him. I knelt on the asphalt and saw the boy was breathing and miraculously talking. I called for the pediatric backboard, stripped off most of his clothes to look for other injuries, and wrapped him in the many Velcro straps of the board, completely immobilizing him.

He remained conscious and talked to us all the way to the

ER. His mom sat in the seat at the top of the gurney. The boy tried in earnest to move his strapped head so he could see his mom, but only his eyes strained upward.

He said to her, "Hi, Mom, what are you doing here? Where am I?" Then his eyes would strain to the left and ask me, "What happened? Where's my skateboard?"

After handing him over the ER staff and cleaning up the ambulance, I sat in the nurses' station and began my paperwork.

My preceptor caught me staring at the wall and asked, "Are you okay?"

I broke from my daydream and said, "Oh ya, I'm fine. I thought that call went well." I focused back on finishing my paperwork. We then headed out, ready to run another call.

My journey as a shit magnet had begun. Then and for years to come, I seemed to get the gnarliest calls. And yet I couldn't have been happier. I was blissfully unaware of how much I was asking the box in my head to hold.

In May 1991, I'd completed the 480 hours of riding third on the ambulance and being watched, critiqued, and encouraged. I'd had a few stern talking-tos and experienced having a team of people who always had my back. I passed all my tests and got my blue card in the mail, saying I was a licensed paramedic. It happened so fast I had only two days off between finishing my internship and starting as a paramedic.

I couldn't wait to get started, even though the self-doubting loner in me was afraid of making a mistake. Now I worked on my own. I would have an EMT partner, and I would be the only paramedic on scene, unless we needed another ambulance for multiple patients. If my EMT partner screwed up, it would be my responsibility.

~

That summer I worked full-time, making $6.25 an hour. I enrolled in a few classes at UC Davis for the fall, planning to cut back on my hours at work once school started—but that never happened.

CHAPTER FIVE

I drove to Fairfield to work a Saturday shift. The bright sun and clear blue sky made for a beautiful day, and I was eager to run some calls. In the afternoon, we were dispatched to a suicide attempt. I was still a new medic, but I'd already been on a handful of these calls.

We pulled up to a nicely landscaped house, with a Fairfield fire engine already on scene. We hopped out of the ambulance and hurriedly grabbed our equipment. A police officer directed us through a wooden side gate and into the backyard. A middle-aged man in jeans and a plaid shirt sat in a chair. The man had put a shotgun in his mouth and pulled the trigger. The image before me was straight out of a horror movie.

The energy we had rushing through the gate drained as we processed what we saw. Three silent Fairfield firefighters sat with slumped postures on the edge of a planter with tears in their eyes.

"That's our captain," one of them said.

I didn't know what to think or say. All I could come up with was, "So sorry for your loss."

I couldn't relate to this man. I was so thrilled with my life; things couldn't get any better. Many years from this day, I would arrive at the same stage of my career, and I, too, would put a gun in my mouth and contemplate pulling the trigger. But for now, I was in love with this job.

With nothing to do, my partner and I picked up our unopened medical bags and left the dead fire captain and his three devastated firefighters.

We then headed to Tacos Jalisco for burritos because it was lunchtime and we were hungry. We'd run a horrific call, and stuff it away so we could go on to the next call. It may sound crazy but that's what we did.

It's what all first responders do.

A physiological response triggers when you're on your way to an emergency. No matter how calm and collected first responders remain, adrenaline courses through our bodies that we must learn how to harness. For me, a ribbon of pure, red-hot energy corkscrews through my core. It starts like a thousand fluttering butterflies in my stomach and then splits off from my center and bores into my legs and arms. A fragment of ribbon reaches up and grabs my vocal cords and plugs my ears. The ribbon can reach its way into my eyes and tunnel my vision.

I believe the skilled and veteran first responders know how to keep this kind of energy out of their eyes, ears, and vocal cords, but it can move too fast for most newbies to control. The ribbon can seize your legs and cause you to run to the engine and move too fast, therefore making mistakes. It can latch onto your vocal cords and make it difficult to talk. It can cover your eyes so that all you can see is the flames. There's much more to the scene in front of you. It can plug your ears so you hear almost nothing. Mastering the ribbon separates those who perform well from those who buckle under the pressure. The bigger the mess, the more furiously the ribbon expands and moves.

Most people think first responders get into the business to help people. The truth is, helping people is just a bonus. I believe most of us do it for the exquisite clarity that comes from mastering the ribbon. It's like a professional athlete being in the zone. From the moment you are dispatched to a fire, a mad race starts to be the first person through the door. If I'm not in the fight, I don't matter, and the ribbon retracts. And since there's no greater feeling than when that red hot ribbon surges through me, followed by the most intense clarity, the letdown of the ribbon retracting is crushing.

I later came to believe I learned to master my ribbon in my childhood. Growing up in all that chaos, I learned to not only function but thrive in such conditions.

This would explain how I managed a call on a late sunny morning in Vallejo. Dispatch had been quiet all morning. After showering, checking out our rigs, and getting our mochas and scones from down the street, we played Nintendo. The dispatch phone rang. We paused the game and answered the phone. They dispatched us to a house fire three blocks away.

Before the garage doors rolled up, we heard the fire department sirens and air horns pounding in the distance. I could feel the extra urgency of the fire department. My body reacted, and we were on our way.

Once we arrived on the scene, I located the incident commander. Pressurized flames blew out of every second-story window of the house. In the street, a screaming and sobbing woman grabbed onto a firefighter begging him to save her babies. That firefighter's job was to operate the pump panel on the fire engine to deliver water through the fire hoses, so he kept pushing her away, pleading with her.

"We are! You have to let go of me so I can do my job!"

As a police officer peeled the hysterical mother off of him, her upper body leaned forward, and her arms remain outstretched toward the firefighter screaming "Please!"

As the police tried to contain the mother, I got close to her face. I made eye contact with her, and she quieted, looking into my eyes, searching for something to grab onto. I asked her how many kids were inside.

She screamed, "Fooouuur!"

We were going to need more ambulances. I quickly radioed dispatch to send me three more. By myself, there was no way I could help four kids if this looked to be as bad as it was.

Just as I finished keying the radio mic, a firefighter exited the front door of the house and said to me, "I need you to come inside and check on this kid we brought down from the second floor, to see if there is anything you can do."

"You can't bring him out?"

The firefighter gave me a two-second stare, as if his brain was searching for an answer. The mother was nowhere in sight, and therefore out of mind. Still, I waited for him to find the words. "No," he said, "You need to come inside."

"Is it safe?" I asked

He nodded. "The fire's contained to the second floor."

I followed him through the front door into the uninvolved first floor. In the middle of a normal, unaffected living room, a charred and blackened figure lay on his back on beige carpet. His legs and arms were bent and stiff in the air as if he'd been flash frozen while kneeling on all fours. This child wasn't flash frozen, just burned beyond recognition. Fire had consumed his ears, hands, face, and toes.

The firefighter and I locked eyes for a moment as now I searched for something to say. All I found was, "Leave this inside." *No one needs to see this kid or what's left of him.*

I exited the front door and walked out into the street. Ten steps later, I saw a different firefighter exit the house holding a bundle, limp little legs softly bouncing with each hurried step the firefighter took. His turnouts were covered in black charcoal marks and his sweaty face showed a heavy trail of black soot that began at his upper lip and right into his nostrils. He'd taken off his own air mask during the fire and in the thick smoke to put over the face of this little kid. He handed her over to me. She couldn't have been more than three years old.

As soon as she was in my arms, the firefighter put his self-contained breathing apparatus (SCBA) mask back on and disappeared into the house again, rushing back into the second-story inferno.

The girl lay limp, and gray skin hung off of her like spider webbing. Only a handful of blond curls remained on the back of her head. Her face was dark and burned. She was breathing, but barely. I headed toward the open back doors of my ambulance, stepped up the back step, and laid her down on a blue burn sheet. I grabbed my airway kit and my partner bagged the little girl, a process that involves blowing air into the lungs with a bag valve mask.

I immediately heard more commotion behind me and stepped down the back steps of the ambulance. My eyes locked on another firefighter headed toward me with the same trail of soot under his nose, this time carrying an infant. I hurriedly met him in the middle of the street and took an even smaller child, this one maybe a one-year-old. Skin hung off the baby boy who struggled to breathe.

I put him on my gurney next to his sister. Then again, before I knew it, the same goddamned thing. Another dirty, unmasked firefighter, another burned, barely breathing kid had been dug out of the second floor of that house. I ran to meet him and took the third child into my arms, this child about two years old. I had three kids barely clinging to life and only one of me.

Mercifully, another ambulance pulled up before I got to the back of mine. Mike, a paramedic I'd worked closely with for a while, jumped out and shouted, "Christy!"

The second I saw him, I handed off the child I carried like a football. All I said to him was, "Go! I don't have a destination for you," meaning he needed to get the kid to one of the two nearby hospitals.

As I swung my head back around, my eyes saw the mother in the back of a police car. There was no more yelling or sobbing. She sat almost comatose, her eyes open and staring, her head slumped against the window. I climbed into my ambulance to attend to two of her barely breathing kids. *What the fuck!* traveled through my head. We were about to leave for the hospital with both kids when the third ambulance arrived. Another medic I worked with and knew well jumped into my ambulance and grabbed the two-year-old.

Now I had one child to attend to on the way to the hospital. A firefighter shut the rear ambulance doors and another one jumped up front to drive so my partner and I could slip a teeny tiny breathing tube into the baby's teeny tiny trachea. This should have happened immediately, but there were too many children to tend to. Everything had happened in a matter of minutes rather than the fucking eternity it felt like.

A few days after the fire, my partner and I arrived at Children's Hospital in Oakland due to an unrelated call. While we were there, we wanted to visit the kids from the fire. We made the trek upstairs to the ICU and somewhat proudly told the nurses at the front desk we were the medics who'd taken care of those kids at the fire.

She walked us to the room with two of the three kids, mummies in their beds. Their entire bodies, even their faces and heads, were wrapped in gauze. Tubes came out of everywhere. Both lay on their backs with their arms and legs spread-eagle, just like they had on my gurney. Their fresh pink burns had turned swollen, gnarled, and angry-red with blood and pus leaking through the gauze. Their condition shocked me and my partner. I didn't know why we expected anything different; we knew the treatment for severe burns. Both burns and road rash looked their "best" right when they happen. The body's healing response transformed the wounds into horrible factories of pain and gruesome bodily detritus.

As I walked away, I thought of how they wouldn't feel love or comfort from being held, if they even survived. The suffering they experienced was unimaginable. I wondered if sometimes we caused more harm than good by saving a life.

A few weeks later, I attended the critical incident stress debriefing for that fire. I sat in a circle of folding chairs amongst all the others involved—paramedics, EMTs, firefighters, ER nurses, flight nurses, and doctors outwardly expressed some form of grief. Many cried, having difficulty speaking, and even the old dinosaur firefighters had tears in their eyes. A few firefighters fidgeted in their chairs and when their turn came, they said they didn't want to talk, even though they were visibly affected. They said there were people in the room they didn't trust.

In the circle of first responders, everyone showed signs of being affected except for me. I wasn't trying to hold anything back. My brain desperately worked to manufacture some tears so I wouldn't look like a heartless asshole, but the tears, difficulty talking, or grief never came. I talked about a bunch of burned kids and a mom like I was describing a trip to the grocery store. From the moment I heard the emphatic wail of the fire department's sirens and the pounding of their air horns, my brain had stuffed each moment of that call into the box in my mind, including the children and the mom.

By the end of the call, I'd closed the lid.

CHAPTER SIX

I learned to drink coffee at this job. I worked 96–120 hours a week, as did most of us. There were always extra shifts needing to be filled, and I could not get enough. I loved this job and it loved me. Controlling the ribbon brought me clarity and fulfillment. However, the amount of gritty, gnarly calls I responded to continued to grow.

On May 9, 1995, we responded to a head-on collision on Highway 37 in Vallejo. The speed limit on this highway was fifty-five, but no one heeded the limit. We arrived on scene prior to the fire department and found a sedan with the front end completely smashed in. Another vehicle, a white sedan rested about forty feet from the first car. Its front end was also crumpled to the windshield. The driver's door hung open; the seatbelt hung in the door. A woman lay crumpled on the ground several feet from her car. She had been ejected and landed on the shoulder of the road. It was clear she hadn't been wearing the lap belt.

I walked to the car with the driver inside. His face and body looked intact, but he was dead, his face drained of all color. The impact and sudden deceleration of his body had ripped his internal organs from their functional places.

I said to the CHP officer, "He's dead," and turned toward the woman on the side of the road.

"He's a cop," the officer said.

I paused a millisecond before moving to the woman. She had a heart rhythm but no pulse. This meant the electricity in her heart still fired, but the heart remained still. I had my airway bag out and intubated her on the road. My partner performed CPR. I put the tube down her throat and into her lungs and started an IV. We did CPR and I gave the woman first-round cardiac drugs, epinephrine and atropine. I told my partner to stop chest compression so we could check the EKG he'd hooked up before he had started the CPR. A few more electrical beats danced across the screen but became farther and farther spaced out until a flat green line moved silently across the screen. She died right in front of me.

We'd raced to the scene, engaged all of ourselves to keep these people alive, and now it was over. We cleaned up our stuff, took the woman off the EKG monitor, and I completed my patient care reports for the coroner. I asked CHP if they needed anything else, got back into our ambulance, then headed back into downtown Vallejo.

As we entered the city limits and radioed our availability, we were dispatched to a cancer patient with difficulty breathing. We turned the red lights and siren back on. Once again, we engaged ourselves to save a life.

We arrived at the house and carried the same bags we'd just put away. A man with tears in his eyes met us at the front door and directed us upstairs to a bedroom. We walked past several more people with tears in their eyes. They surrounded a woman, her body flaccid, lying in bed. She wore a red-and-orange scarf on her head, the sign of a cancer patient. Her head rested to the side, her mouth open in the shape of an O. Everyone understood she was dying. I faced her grieving family.

"What can we do for you all?"

"She's on Hospice care," the man who'd greeted me at the door said. "We didn't know what to do."

"Have you called hospice?"

"Yes, we did."

"Does she have a do-not-resuscitate order?"

"No, she doesn't."

"Do you want her to go to the hospital?"

"No! We want her home."

This put us in a sticky situation. Since she didn't have a DNR, legally we couldn't just leave her to die in peace with her family. Yet, since she was in hospice, dying of a terminal illness, I could not bring myself to drag her into the hospital, away from her family and comfortable surroundings. She deserved to die at home.

I called the emergency room on a recorded radio channel to get approval not to transport her, since paramedics work under a doctor's standing orders. There were some situations requiring us to get permission. I explained our situation with the nurse, and we discussed our options.

The nurse finally said, "I guess you're going to have to stay there until she dies."

"What?"

"Well, legally if you leave now that's abandonment. The doctor agrees bringing her to the hospital would only be harder on her and the family, so the only choice we have is for you to stay until she dies and then turn the deceased over to the coroner."

So we stayed. We stayed in the room, surrounded by the family in their most intimate moments of saying goodbye. For an hour, her heart slowly quieted until the green line moved in a straight line across the monitor.

When she was gone, we radioed the police, which is standard procedure, and they officially released the beloved family member's body to the family to be taken to the funeral home rather than to the coroner. My partner and I took the woman off the monitor, expressed our condolences, and left. Again, we walked away with nothing but death and emptiness.

As we drove back to the station, we passed a flatbed tow truck carrying the crumpled cars we'd seen earlier on Highway 37. My partner and I just exchanged a quick glance. *You gotta be fucking kidding me.*

CHAPTER SEVEN

In December 1995, my friend Judy invited me to a Professional Women's Club night at a local gay bar. I was reluctant to go—bars weren't my thing, I was not a professional and therefore didn't belong—but she talked me into it. I had just recently been dumped from a three-year relationship and wanted to feel sorry for myself for a little while longer. But once I arrived, I worked the group with jokes and banter. The attention from the women filled me with energy and hope.

One woman walked in late to the group, coming from playing in a softball game. She introduced herself as Lisa and sat down at our table. She was cute and had an amazing smile but rarely made eye contact. She seemed quiet and shy, and I was determined to get a reaction from her. I directed my jokes and banter toward her, hoping to engaged her. She laughed at me in that "courtesy laugh" way.

After about an hour and a half, Lisa stood up and said, "Well, I'm leaving and going home. I'm cold."

"Stay," I said.

"I would, but I really am cold," she said.

"If you dance with me, I'll warm you up." I was flirting.

She looked down at the floor, "Ya thanks, but that won't work."

The room wasn't remotely cold, so I let her go, figuring I

would not be able to wrangle her attention. When she left, I continued to talk to the group.

The next week, Judy called me. "Lisa, the woman at the bar . . . she likes you." Judy gave me Lisa's number. "You need to call her."

"Yeah, right," I said, doubting Lisa's sincerity. "She totally blew me off. Plus, I don't want to go out with anyone right now." I just got out of a three-year relationship that ended poorly. "I'm pretty happy just being on my own."

But Judy pestered me for a month, relentlessly telling me to call her.

I finally said, "If I call her, will you stop harassing me?"

Judy agreed.

I called, got an answering machine, and left a message. I never heard back.

For another two weeks, Judy still harassed me to call Lisa again. So, I called her again to get Judy off my back. This time, Lisa answered the phone and we talked for almost an hour. Then she invited me over for a small gathering at her house.

Eight years older than me, Lisa drove a spotless, white Volvo station wagon and had an amazing smile. Everything about her was sensible—even her PTA-style, mom haircut. Her house was very organized and tidy. She showed up to every appointment early and never procrastinated. I always procrastinated and was always late back then. (Now I am never late.) Everything she did was thought out and planned for. I preferred to fly by the seat of my pants.

Lisa had grown up on an agricultural farm in Fresno. She learned planning was a must because even when everything was great, an insect or bad weather could wipe out an entire crop.

Where I loved dogs and kids, Lisa loved cats and had no idea how to relate to a kid. Growing up on a farm, she never really got to be one herself. I was failing classes at UC Davis, and she had graduated from UC Davis and then attended graduate school and received her MBA. I loved to cook, and she used her oven for storage. The sight of blood made her faint, and I couldn't get enough of it. And where I was always hot, she was always cold. She really wasn't blowing me off when we first met.

We seemed to be complete opposites—she an introvert and me an extrovert—but my playfulness and lack of worry was attractive to her, and her stability and security was attractive to me.

As friends of ours would later say, "What one isn't good at, the other one is."

During the small party she hosted at her house, I had a great time hanging out with her friends. I barely talked to Lisa, as she was busy being hostess. But I thought if these were the people she surrounded herself with, she had to be good.

We continued seeing each other, but I was not ready to rush into anything. I had been cheated on and lied to in my previous relationship. A friend from work and I rented a house in Crockett. I wanted some time, and a space to call my own. Lisa was patient and understood and never nagged me about it. In fact, she never nagged me about anything. I'd do twenty-four, forty-eight, seventy-two, and ninety-six-hour shifts. I'd have to cancel plans because I got stuck at work or I'd be too exhausted from working for two days straight.

A paramedic's schedule was hard on a couple. Lisa had a normal job working Monday through Friday, eight to five, and I worked twenty-four-hour shifts. She'd sleep in on Saturdays and my alarm would sound off early for work. I came home Sunday mornings exhausted or sometimes not at all. I'd finally get a Saturday off and a bunch of my friends had included me in their plans.

Sometimes I would ask myself in this situation, *Should I have stayed home and spent time with Lisa or gone out with my friends?* The extreme introvert in Lisa kept her from going with me to see my friends; but if I never saw my friends, I wouldn't have any friends.

Whatever I did, I was always letting someone else down. This was hard for me, since I based my self-worth on making everyone happy. But I was also falling deeply in love with Lisa, so the stress seemed worth it.

After we'd been serious for about a year, I believed this relationship had a future and moved in with Lisa. She cleared out a second room for me to put my stuff in and have my own little space. I came with few belongings, so there was no having to mix furniture. We took down the weird wallpaper, and she painted the room.

I came home from work one morning and I looked at my freshly painted room. "Thank you so much . . . but . . . it's pink."

"Shit, you are right. I don't know how that happened. That's not the color I picked out. I am going to repaint it."

And she did.

CHAPTER EIGHT

I loved working with Vallejo Fire. All the firefighters were kind, good at their jobs, and always wanted to help. The Vallejo Fire Department did not have paramedics, so no one was there to help me with those skills, but they had a tremendous amount of experience and always had my back.

When someone calls 911 for a medical emergency, a fire engine and an ambulance are sent. Many people ask why is that necessary for a medical call. Well, when a 250-pound naked person has had a major heart attack and has fallen between the toilet and the wall, and their house is on the third floor with no elevator, it takes more than two people to handle the situation. And this happens quite often.

Watching firefighters perform their job made me want to be one of them. In 1996, around the time I moved in with Lisa, I decided to attend an eighteen-week fire academy at the Solano Community College to get my Firefighter I Certificate.

I loved everything about it. I loved getting dirty and smelling like smoke and physically pushing myself. The day I entered a burning building for the first time, we knelt just outside the door so when the instructor opened it, we would be below the heat. When he opened the door, a whoosh of heat came at and over us. As we went through the door crawling on our knees to stay below the high heat, we dragged the hose line down a hallway.

A voice inside my head quietly said, "Ummm you are not supposed to go in there." A much louder voice yelled, "Let's go! This is so cool!" The "ribbon" surged through my body at a heightened level I had never felt before. The thrill of this experience took my taming of the ribbon to a new level. Not just another person's life was in my hands, but now my own life was on the line.

I wanted to be a firefighter so badly, I was willing to work as hard as I had to. The first physical agility test I took kicked my ass, so I went to the gym and lifted weights. I had trouble with the oral interviews, so I worked on my posture and professionalism.

Even with all that work, it took me three years of testing at several fire departments in the greater Bay Area to be hired.

The firefighter job I finally landed started in a sea of tables and three hundred twenty-somethings in T-shirts and baseball hats. An older man, standing at the front, grabbed his reading glasses that hung around his neck and put them on his face. He looked over the top of them, hoping the room would get a clue and shut up.

He said, "Welcome to the Contra Costa County Fire Protection District firefighter's written test. There are forty-five hundred people taking this test today."

I stopped listening and almost got up and left. There was no question of passing the test. They were all the same and I had taken quite a few. But my chances of getting a job out of this giant pool of people were slim. And I was not more likely to get a job just because I was a woman.

Despite my pessimism, I stayed for the tests. After passing the physical agility test and the oral board interviews, I went in for a chief's interview.

Four white men wearing fancy class A uniforms covered in gold accessories sat across the table from me in the interview room. They smiled as I shook each one of their hands, and then they invited me to sit down. They asked all the questions I had heard before. At the end of the interview, they asked if there was anything else I would like to add. I had a few lines in store for these moments—about how if you hire me, I won't let you down, and bla-bla-bla, but something else fell out of my mouth this time.

"I know I don't look like a big, strong firefighter," I said, "but I promise you, I can do the work of a big strong firefighter, and I have the heart of one, too."

I stood up and we all shook hands again. I walked out of there thinking, *I either just totally blew it or caught their attention.*

A few weeks later, on May 19, 1997, a nice lady called to offer me a job with the Moraga Fire District, a department that shared an administration with Contra Costa Fire.

I let out a piercing scream in the nice lady's ear.

The job came with a seventeen-week academy run by the Contra Costa County Fire Protection District (CCCFPD). The academy consisted of recruits from CCCFPD, Moraga Fire, and Orinda Fire Department. After surviving the first week, all of us in the academy decided to celebrate. A bunch of the guys wanted to shave their heads, so we had a beer and head-shaving party.

I shaved Matt Burton's head. I had known Matt for a while since we'd gone through the reserve academy together, and I'd always liked him. He had also been a reserve for CCCFPD, and this was his dream job. He was strong and smart and like me, and would never stop until he became a firefighter. All of us in the fire academy bonded and worked hard together. We learned how to throw ladders (put ladders up) and how to pull and flake out hose to quickly pull it into and through a structure. We learned how to cut four- by eight-foot holes in a pitched roof with axes and chain saws. They taught us to build rope systems to rescue a person off a cliff or a building and to repel down the five-story drill tower. We had days we felt strong and confident, and days we struggled and felt defeated.

After seventeen long weeks, graduation day came and I finally put on that wool uniform. I received a real badge and a red sticker for my car that let everyone know I was a firefighter. I believed I had moved up in the world and was now part of an elite group. Only the toughest become firefighters, and I was one of them.

My first day on duty with the Moraga-Orinda Fire Department (MOFD), at Station 41, I walked through the open apparatus bay carrying my turnouts, and a kind firefighter introduced himself. He showed me where to put my gear and introduced me to the two paramedics I would be assigned to during the five-call evaluation process. And then, they handed me a mop. Rather than be offended by this, I was thankful to have something to do instead of standing around nervously.

From my first day, I heard grumblings around the department regarding the previous woman who had worked at MOFD. She developed a poor reputation because of her lack of ability to do the job and get along with others. As soon as I arrived, I was measured in comparison to this other firefighter simply because we were both women.

Working twice as hard to prove myself because of my gender was not new to me.

Since MOFD provided fire, rescue, and paramedic services to a sleepy, affluent, bedroom town with little commercial property, we didn't run many calls. Of course, some days we were busy, and the emergency rooms were far away, but mostly we spent our time on station and equipment maintenance, public service demonstrations, and training.

One day, our battalion chief set up a lost firefighter drill. One of our guys in full gear hid somewhere in the darkened building. It was our job to find him and get him out. We all wore our full gear, too, and breathed through our SCBA.

This was no game of hide-and-seek; we had a thought-out plan for finding the missing firefighter, staying together, and not getting lost ourselves. I entered the building and started with a right-hand search. I got lucky and found our victim quickly, but he was also under some crap and surrounded by more crap.

On my own, I moved the big stuff out of the way and dragged him over the small stuff, out of the building and into the parking lot to where our battalion chief stood.

I let go of the firefighter's SCBA strap, pulled off my helmet and mask and said, "Who says women don't belong in the fire service?" and gave a stern look.

My BC quietly and hesitantly said, "I never said that."

It was true; he hadn't. He hired me, but, as usual, I had everything to prove.

About six months later, a captain and I sat on the engine's tailboard waiting for the driver.   Making small talk, he said, "So I am hearing good things about you."

"Really?" My insides beamed. I knew I was good at my job, but I didn't know what everyone thought. This validation from guys in a fire department allowed me to take a deep breath.

"Yeah. People are saying you're an excellent paramedic and you can hold your own on the fireground. Many of us were leery when we heard they hired a woman."

"Well, thank you for telling me. That's nice."

"Although, you know most women in the fire service don't

make it to full retirement. They tend to get hurt or move to a desk job."

"Not me," I said. "No way in hell. Unless something catastrophic happens, I will make it to retirement." He meant no ill will; he was just stating what's statistically true. I promised myself I would not be that woman. I would make it until retirement, no matter what it took.

This vow planted itself in the back of my head and became a permanent fixture.

A few weeks later, the alarm blasted at 2:00 a.m., and the room instantaneously burst with light. I put my legs into my boots and my red suspenders over my shoulders. We suited up, climbed into the engine, and headed out while I shook the sleep from my eyes. We pulled up to a multiple-story apartment building, which I saw immediately housed seniors. Our battalion chief showed up behind us. I headed in alongside my captain and battalion chief and opened the door to the third-floor hallway. It was like stepping into another universe. Smoke filled the hallways, as did elderly men and women aimlessly wandering around. The lights stayed on so I would see a person disappear into the smoke and another one emerge. It was like a scene from a zombie movie.

As we made our way down the hallway to the apartment on fire, a resident shouted, "There's still someone in there!"

We quickly dashed into the apartment. My captain and chief went left, and I went right, into the bedroom. I crawled on my hands and knees, searching the room. I crawled between the far wall and the bed. A woman's ashen face popped out of the smoke like a clown in a fun house, scaring the shit out of me.

"I got one!" I yelled to my captain. As soon as those words came out of my mouth, I couldn't believe it. I sounded like Billy McCaffrey in *Backdraft* when he found his first fire victim. What a tool I was. But the thought quickly disappeared because a burned woman lay in front of me, barely breathing.

Within seconds, my captain was by my side. I picked her up from under the shoulders and he picked up her legs. We carried her down the long hallway, through the maze of zombie residents, and waited for the elevator, where it was safe to take the elevator and much quicker. I walked into the elevator backward and leaned against the back wall, still holding the woman. Time stood still, and my brain threw up a giant red flag. *What are you doing?*

In my previous life as a paramedic, a firefighter would have carried the person out, and I, the paramedic, would be the one to put the victim on a sterile burn sheet on the gurney. I would have handled the person delicately.

Now as a firefighter, my role was to get her out of the hazardous area. While in the elevator, I realized my turnouts were ripping burned skin off of her as I held her.

The elevator doors opened into a bright and clean lobby filled with residents waiting out the incident. Bored faces turned to horrified faces. Angry remorse hit me as we exposed all these people to their burned neighbor. We hurriedly headed out of the lobby, through the entrance to where an ambulance was backing up.

We held the woman in the same position while the medics jumped out, tore the gurney out, and placed the blue burn sheet on it lightning fast. My arms began to cramp, and I was grateful to put the woman down. I stepped back as the medics took over. I looked down at my front side and saw how much of the woman remained on my coat. *Do I brush her skin off, right here, onto the parking lot asphalt?*

My captain's voice pulled me from my discord. "We gotta go plug that sprinkler head," he said.

I walked to the engine, pretending there wasn't a person's skin all over the front of me. I put the entire experience in the box and closed the lid. I grabbed the sprinkler kit and headed back up to the third floor.

We were up the rest of the night doing overhaul and waiting for the fire marshal to arrive and complete her investigation. Once back at the station, I had one hour before it was time to go home. I took off my turnouts and left them in a tangled pile on the floor. Normally I would take care of that myself, since the turnouts had an inner and outer layer that had to be separated in addition to closing all the clasps and buttons. My body repelled away from watching pieces of the woman's skin float to the floor, so I asked the oncoming crew to toss them in the washer.

That night taught me the smell of burned human skin coats the inside of your nose and sinuses for several days.

MOFD was a great department to work for. My battalion chief was one of the best human beings I knew. He was a hell of a firefighter and fire ground leader. The paramedics were extremely good. They treated me as part of the team. But I missed running a lot of calls. Moraga and Orinda were quiet communities, and I liked and needed to be busy. I craved the days in Vallejo where we would respond to call after call after call. I even missed being up all night and going home exhausted, but full of satisfaction and contentment. At MOFD, we mostly slept at night, with an occasional call to interrupt whatever community service or education we were doing. We had our critical calls and fires, but they just didn't come at a furious pace.

I had tested at Berkeley prior to getting hired at MOFD, and I was on their hiring list. Finally, they called me in for a chief's interview.

CHAPTER NINE

When I got the Berkeley job, I let out a happy scream followed by some fist pumps.

I had loved my time at MOFD, but Berkeley had lots of action—old, non-fireproof construction, poorly behaved people, and target hazards, such as a building posing a great danger. And our acronym was BFD. How much better could it get?

Working for the Berkeley Fire Department was going to solve a problem that had long plagued me. I'd finally be someone who mattered. I would be someone special who stood above the average throngs and who belonged to something exclusive. Only the best of the best got hired to BFD.

Captain Williams stated it to us new hires during orientation at family day. "You ten are the cream of the crop."

I couldn't wait to work my ass off, test myself, push myself, and be part of a smart, hardworking, cohesive team. Fire academies pushed and tested a person's limits. The job mattered, and it mattered that it was done well. A person succeeded or failed. By completing a tough and demanding academy, I would prove I belonged there.

Fire departments start new hires from the beginning, as if they know nothing about firefighting. Each fire department has their own way of accomplishing tasks, and they have different equipment. Different departments carry different length ladders and have different ways of throwing them.

The goal of the academy was to learn and practice a skill repeatedly until a firefighter built muscle memory to avoid having to think about it. We had to be able to perform those skills at 3:00 a.m., after being ripped out of sleep, heart racing and chaos storming.

When the academy began, I spent twelve weeks learning different ways to load and pull hose, throw ladders, and become an expert in using new tools, saws, and equipment. I also memorized different emergency medical protocols, new streets, and new policies. As always, I worked as hard as possible to never show any weakness.

As a female firefighter, weakness can't be even a fleeting thought. If a male firefighter goes down in a fire, people will say and think, "Wow, what a hero! He wasn't afraid to put himself in harm's way to get the job done." If a female firefighter goes down, those same people think and say, "She should have never been there in the first place. She couldn't handle the job." This is just one of the double standards women in this line of work face.

I was determined to prove myself capable and strong.

Graduation day finally came. My entire family was there. My dad came down from Oregon, my brother came up from LA, and my mom came from Palo Alto. The graduates stood at the front of the room. Part of the ceremony included all of us being sworn in and then receiving our badges, designating we were sworn members of the fire department. We swore to protect people, property, and the environment. We swore to be courageous. We swore to do our jobs with integrity. The swearing in and badge allowed firefighters to go places citizens and the unsworn could not go.

Tradition decreed that firefighters choose someone to pin their badge on them. I chose my mom. Even though my mom wasn't there for me when I was growing up, she taught me I could be whatever I wanted to be. She would tell me to not let anyone or anything stop me. From her I learned anything was possible. The world was mine.

Growing up, the only firefighters or paramedics I ever saw were male. I didn't even know a woman could be one. After becoming a paramedic, I realized I could be a firefighter, and now that I'd achieved it, I knew I could be whatever I wanted, provided I could do the job well.

I got out of the academy and was assigned to Station Two. Since the academy left me wanting more, I looked forward to getting out in the field. For the first six months, they assigned each new firefighter to a captain. I hoped for a salty guy who would push me and give me opportunities to rise to the challenge. And I really hoped to be judged on merit.

My disappointment with the department's lack of standards and discipline was palpable from the first day. The morning I got off duty from my first day at BFD, another of my academy mates was coming on duty. He pulled me aside so no one could hear and said, "Hey Christy, can I borrow your flash hood? I forgot mine at home."

I gave him my flash hood but immediately judged him. I thought, *How in the fuck do you forget your flash hood on your first day?* We had just gotten out of the academy, and the expectations were so clear. Plus, this guy used to be the chief of another department. He was our golden boy—smart, muscular, and handsome. I knew that if I'd forgotten my flash hood, I never would have heard the end of it, and I would have been just as hard on myself.

For the next six months, I was assigned to work under Captain Brown at Station 2. He was six foot five, strong, and powerful. I had no doubt he could pick up a small car and throw it. When I first met him, I immediately sensed his kindness and gentleness. I felt some relief as I knew immediately I would not have to deal with any "female firefighter" bullshit. But over time, as I got to know him, I realized he would not challenge me in the ways I'd hoped to be challenged. I was desperate to prove myself.

On one of my shifts assigned to Station 2, I was on Medic 2, one of our three ambulances. The darkness of the late evening had fallen. Medic 2 and Engine 2 were dispatched to a shooting with BPD on scene. We arrived and a twenty-two-year-old male lay on the ground. He had been shot in the back, just under his left shoulder blade.

He writhed around in pain screaming, "Help me!"

Since he had a gunshot to the chest, we had to move fast. He needed a surgeon, not us. My partner and I quickly picked him up and put him on a backboard. We got him into the ambulance as fast as we could. As I leaned over him to access the EKG monitor on the shelf on the other side of him, he reached up and grabbed my shirt. His dark brown eyes opened wide with terror and locked onto mine.

Between his rapid breaths for air, he pleaded, "Don't let me die. Oh my God. Please don't let me die."

"I'm doing everything I can, but you gotta let go of me."

He didn't let go, so I pulled one of his hands from the grip he had on my shirt, and his other hand followed.

I would never promise anyone they were not going to die. Lying at a moment like this would be to rob a person of whatever experience unfolds before they die. A bullet had just ripped through this guy's chest, so I knew his chances were slim. But if I could just get him to the emergency room alive, he might have a chance.

His writhing slowed while his breathing rate increased. The amount of air he moved in and out of his lungs became less and less until he breathed like a fish out of water. I stuck a large needle into his chest, hoping to relieve the pressure inside, but blood came streaming out instead of air. I stuck another large needle into the other side of his chest. I was grateful when air came out of that side. His breathing rate decreased and continued to until it stopped. I quickly intubated him and just as we pulled into the Highland Hospital Emergency Room parking lot, his heart stopped.

We started CPR and got him inside the ER as fast as we could. As soon as we passed the threshold of the trauma room, I began delivering my verbal report to the doctors, nurses, and ER techs, about twelve people who stood in a circle around the hospital gurney. We awkwardly danced with the staff as we rushed to get us and our gurney out of the way, while most of the staff descended around him like ants to a drop of honey. We moved the gurney to the hallway, came back into the room, and stood near the scribe nurse.

We had a front-row seat to the production. There was someone evaluating each part of the patient. Each evaluator would call out the condition of their particular part to the nurse who scribed. They talked at once and over each other. The new medical students yelled, not yet having learned how to control their ribbon. The trauma surgeon stood at the foot of the bed with his arms folded, taking it all in. The nurses started IVs and gave him fluid and blood. They continued CPR. An X-ray technician rolled his large portable machine in and took a chest X-ray.

The choreographed mayhem lasted for about ten minutes

until the trauma surgeon, who was in charge, announced, "We aren't getting any response. Let's crack his chest."

I watched while a couple of nurses grabbed some instruments and poured iodine all over the kid's chest. The surgeon cut open his chest and exposed the guy's completely still heart. He stuck his hand right into the man's chest and squeezed, manually pumping his heart, but the bullet had torn through the contents of his chest.

After about a minute, the doctor pronounced the twenty-two-year-old dead and called out a time of death. The doctor walked to the garbage can in the room as he was peeling off his blood-soaked gloves.

"Was there anything else I could have done?" I asked.

"Not a thing," he said. "That bullet bounced around like a pin-ball in his chest. It took out everything. Nothing could have saved him." He walked to the sink, washed his hands, grabbed another patient's chart, and went about his rounds.

I already knew there was nothing I could have done, but I needed to quiet my inner critic. I had hoped hearing the answer from the doctor would bring me some relief, but it didn't. My pompous ass of an inner critic was always sure I could do better.

The show was over, and we needed to get back to our ambulance and onto the next call. My partner cleaned the back of the ambulance while I did paperwork. Once we finished, we drove back to Berkeley. A police officer would soon head to the family of the guy to make a death notification.

The twenty-two-year-old kid spent the last minutes of his life with me—a stranger pulling his hands off his desperate effort to cling to something. He looked me straight in the eyes and begged me not to let him die. Who was I to take up the last moments of someone's life like that? Who was I to wash someone's blood off my hands or arms or face straight down the drain? I had never felt worthy to be a part of these kinds of sacred last moments, but I also marveled at the way they transcended the chaos and at how present I always felt.

Near the end of my first six months working with Captain Brown, my expectations for fulfillment at BFD continued to flounder. I loved my captain as a person, but he required little of me. He never challenged me. He'd tell me I was doing fine and that I knew what I was doing. I wanted to train, but my captain only wanted to talk about training.

A requirement of passing probation was to complete our sign-off book. Listed in this book were hose drills, ladder drills, tools, equipment, and knowledge we had to perform or demonstrate. For example, there was a drill that involved carrying an unconscious person down a ladder. I eagerly wanted to perform this task so my coworkers would never doubt whether I had the strength and technique to pull it off.

I approached my captain one shift, a couple months into the job, and asked, "Hey Capt, can I complete this rescue sign off today?"

"Aww, you don't need to do it," he said, "we can just talk about it and that will be enough."

Many of my sign offs played out the same way. My frustration at being held back and not being able to prove my mettle quickly boiled over. I could not believe the department would let anyone pass their probation without proving they could perform all the tasks required to be a solid firefighter. I needed everyone to know without a doubt that I could do the job. If they could see me perform, and if even the salty older guys said I could do the job and vouch for me, I might finally hold value to someone.

Growing up feeling like not even my mother loved me had left me with a deep hole I was constantly trying to fill. I needed to matter to someone . . . to be special to someone. I'd spent my entire life chasing this feeling. When I played sports, I needed to be the best person on the team. With my family and friends, I took care of everyone else, always putting their needs first. I needed to hear people say, "I don't know what I'd do without Christy."

My emotions lived coiled on the surface of every part of me. They sprang into reaction immediately without allowing my brain to process whatever insult they suspected was thrown their way.

Being a firefighter was a perfect job for me because it filled that hole. It gave me something to strive for and my role meant I mattered. But it wasn't enough to just wear the uniform. I wanted to be part of the best of the best. I needed to be the one about whom other firefighters said, "I want Christy on my crew."

Since I didn't get to prove myself during training, I knew I'd have to do it in the field.

Given all this, it's funny I fell in love with Lisa, since she was quiet and didn't talk about or show her emotions.

One of her best friends once told me, "For the first year of our friendship, I wasn't even sure if Lisa liked me or not."

But as the cliché goes, "Still waters run deep." This was and is Lisa.

She is smart and wise beyond her years. She has a tough and cynical exterior, but her middle is soft, loving, and loyal. We make each other laugh. We always joke we are going to be on the bus to hell together for comments we say to each other to make the other laugh. Occasionally, someone will ask me if Lisa is proud that I am a firefighter.

I answer, "I'm not sure because she never talks about it."

So, when I'd ask Lisa if she was proud, she'd answer, "Of course I am. But I could not care less what you do. I will love you the same."

❧

During my first week on the job, we were dispatched to a typical call, a two-story apartment with no elevator. The patient was too weak to make the walk down the stairs, so she would have to be carried down in a stair chair, which was a chair with handles to allow two to four people to carry someone up and down stairs. We stood the woman up, and she turned and sat in the chair. Several firefighter hands reached in and clasped all the seatbelts to keep her in place on the chair. I pushed my way through all those arms to the more difficult side of the chair—the bottom where there's more weight.

One of the other guys said, "We can use four people to carry her."

There was no way I was going to let someone get in the way of me proving myself.

"No. I got it," I said.

"I am sure you can," he replied, "but let's not get anyone hurt. Let's use four people."

Again, I said, "I'm not gonna get hurt. This is easy."

We argued all the way down the stairs.

A few BFD guys had expressed their feelings about women firefighters to me early in my tenure at the department. On one of my first nights at Station 2, Bob and I sat next to each other at dinner.

Between forkfuls and looking down at his plate, Bob said, "You know, I don't think women belong in the fire service. I just don't think they have the strength to do the job."

I glanced at him, surprised at what he just said and replied, "I'm sorry you feel that way. There are some strong women out there."

His gaze never left his plate while he continued to eat. "Well, ya, but not very many."

I didn't say anything. I just ate my dinner.

About four months later, Bob and I responded to a car fire. Once the fire was extinguished, we needed to get into the engine compartment of the car. The hand lever to the hood burned through, so we were going to have to force it open.

Bob said, "Give me your axe."

"What do you want done?" I said. "I'll do it."

He said back, "Just give it to me. We need to get the hood open."

"You aren't getting my axe," I said. "I'll open it." And I did.

Bob wasn't trying to be a jerk. He truly believed women couldn't be strong enough to do the job. He never treated me poorly or unkindly, he just believed women could be a liability.

Honestly, I couldn't blame him. Firefighting was a physically demanding job and strength was paramount. A six-foot male weighing two hundred pounds had legitimate reason to be concerned when a five-foot-six-inch woman weighing one-fifty was tasked with dragging him out of a building. Or when a heavy hoseline had a significant nozzle reaction and there was doubt a woman was strong enough to drag and hold onto the hoseline. I understood a man's trepidation about hiring women.

But their concern certainly did not provide an acceptable reason not to hire women. I vowed to prove no one needed to have any concern about me. My justification for being on this earth depended on it. If I wasn't valuable to this department, I had no reason to exist.

CHAPTER TEN

After two years on the job at BFD, my brother, Kodi, and his wife moved from Los Angeles to Concord, about ten minutes from my house. My brother and I had been far apart for nineteen years and now we'd have a chance to reconnect.

Shortly after moving to the Bay Area, Kodi and his wife got pregnant. I was so excited about becoming an aunt, especially since Lisa didn't want kids, so I'd never be a parent myself. Here was my opportunity to have a kid to love in my life. Kodi and his wife were excited to have me in their child's life, though I was told I had to demonstrate I could go an hour without swearing before I was going to be allowed to babysit!

They named her Alexis. My mom and I were in the delivery room and witnessed her birth. I fell in love at first sight.

Sunday mornings at the firehouse were take-it-easy days. Saturday was the big check-everything-in-the-station day so Sundays could be unstructured. We spent Sundays doing random training, maintenance, or watching football.

One Sunday morning, all of us at Station 5 were tired from being up most of the night. We took a little longer to put on our uniforms and lingered longer at the kitchen table eating breakfast and reading the paper. The thick blanket of fog outside added to the quiet stillness that consumed the morning. The usually constantly ringing station phone stayed quiet. It felt like being in a big city after a snowstorm. The normal noise and bustling was replaced with quiet and empty streets. Finally, we had nothing to pressing to do.

At 9:00 a.m., the dispatch lights and alarm ripped through the stillness and disturbed our quiet morning.

No one moved as we waited to hear dispatch give us the address and nature of the call.

The women's voice through the speakers said, "Engine 2 and Medic 2 respond to XXX Martin Luther King Ave for a baby not breathing. BPD is en route."

Like a magician who snapped his fingers, the relaxed spell was broken, and we hurried to our apparatus, no last quick bite of breakfast or last gulps of coffee.

We pulled up on scene and before the air brakes were even engaged, a Berkeley police officer ran out of the house with a limp baby in his arms. Three of us jumped into the back of the ambulance to receive the hand off from the officer.

"Mom woke up and found him in his crib like this."

My eyes locked on the pattern on his diapers. My niece, who was now two, wore the same ones and was the same age as this kid. Suddenly, instead of an anonymous baby, I saw Alexis, limp on the gurney, blue and not breathing.

Our brains knew this kid was gone, but our hearts didn't want to believe it. Even though we knew for sure he was dead, we still had to do everything we could to save him. This must be done to lessen the burden of failure we'd carry for the rest of our lives. We also did it for the family, so they would know we did everything possible for their child.

One member from the engine crew always rode in the back of ambulance while the other one drove. My job that day was to drive the engine to the hospital to pick up my crew. When the ambulance pulled into the emergency room bay at Children's Hospital Oakland, the medics rushed the baby boy inside. I spotted the Berkeley cop who'd been on the scene as he pulled in right behind us with the baby's mom in the front seat. He took no time parking properly, and he and the mom sprinted into the emergency room.

I didn't go inside, so I started cleaning up the back of the ambulance. When the medics came out a short while later with the now-empty gurney, we stood outside at the back of the ambulance bracing ourselves for the inevitable.

We didn't have to wait long for a scream like no other—the primal kind erupting from the very bottom of a mother's soul.

A firefighter from my engine crew solemnly looked at me and mumbled, "I hate it when I can hear them scream."

Two years went by, and I passed all my probationary tests and requirements. Shortly after, the department began a hiring frenzy.

I felt the quality of paramedic skills of the new hires were not up to par. I grew increasingly frustrated. Berkeley had always hired seasoned medics, and when they hired two new paramedics who'd served in the military as medics, I hoped they'd wow and impress me. Instead, I thought they were terrible paramedics. Some people were in love with them simply because they'd served in the military. While I was extremely grateful for their service to our country, that did not automatically make them good paramedics who should be given a free pass.

I made a big stink that the department should do something about it. I didn't talk behind their backs, either. I told them I thought they sucked right to their faces.

One day I sat at the desk in the station's office and found a patient care report written by one of our new medics. The documentation was lacking, so it appeared the quality of care was lacking. I tossed this at the author of the report and lost it.

"Here! Look at this bullshit! Did you even ask the patient any questions regarding other causes of their chest pain? Did you even ask if they were short of breath?" I ranted on. "Only one fucking blood pressure, one fucking EKG? This is pathetic!" I had absolutely no filter between my brain and my mouth.

He looked at me like, *So, okay, what's your point?*

No one deserved this kind of treatment. What they needed from me was support and mentoring. But I saw everything as being black or white; there was no gray.

My perfectionism was my kryptonite. Everyone should be strong. Everyone should be an excellent paramedic and always respectful. Everyone should clean up after themselves. Everyone should maintain all equipment so that it's spit-shined twenty-four hours a day, three hundred and sixty-five days a year. Even I didn't do that.

A coworker's incompetence made it very possible for my own. If my coworkers weren't the best of the best or even very good at their jobs, what did that say about me? I felt when they fell down on the job, it was a reflection on me because I couldn't be excellent if BFD didn't hire only the best of the best. What if I was only a token female hire?

My need to become a firefighter so I would be a part of the best of the best and feel like I mattered, like I belonged, pulled at me with desperation.

CHAPTER ELEVEN

In 2005, five years into my career at BFD, I was assigned to Engine 6. One midafternoon, my engine and an ambulance from another station were dispatched to an auto vs. pedestrian call. I climbed on the engine and from my designated firefighter's seat. I could only look out the side window. I could not see in front or behind the engine. Until 2008, the rear firefighter seats faced backward—I know, I know, the older guys would say, "and before that we rode on the tailboard."

When I heard the driver say, "Oh no," I knew we were close. I stuck my head out the window and looked toward the front.

A large black-and-white dog, divided in half, lay in the middle of the street. A very similar dog walked around in a circle. An empty school bus sat in the middle of the street.

The engine stopped, and I jumped out. A woman laid on the ground on her side, not moving or making a sound. Blood pooled underneath her head. She looked to be around my age. She wore workout clothes like the kind I wore.

When someone sees something like this, especially since most first responders see so much of it, our brains automatically search for a reason—any reason—not to step into the stream of what is happening and what will happen as news of this person's misery spreads to those who are attached. Sometimes we blame the victim.

Oh, he was drunk off his ass when he plowed into that tree. He brought this on himself. We find some reasoning indicating the person brought it on themselves.

She wasn't wearing her seatbelt. She would have walked away from this if she had.

Or our brains find a way to keep the person distant from us. Anything to make the person different from us, to keep the tragedy and the pain from integrating into ourselves.

This happens somewhere deep in our brains. There is no judgment or treating people differently, it's about self-preservation. Often, we use dark humor. Many on the outside of the paramedic/firefighting world would cringe at what we find humorous. There is no malice or contempt in these jokes, however; it's just survival. These deflection mechanisms will not materialize for a child, however. Our deflection mechanisms are also very hard to summon when we can relate so strongly to someone.

In the case of this woman and her dogs, my survival mechanisms couldn't hold. All three of us on the engine started working on her with our brains upset and our hearts breaking.

The dog who'd survived came over and sat at the woman's head. It just sat still and quiet. The driver of the empty school bus sat on the curb. I glanced at him once and then never did again. I didn't give myself space to think about what must be going through that driver's head. Every molecule of my being focused on the critically injured woman.

About six minutes later, the ambulance showed up with looks on their faces that mirrored ours. The head injury she'd suffered caused her teeth to clench so hard we couldn't get her intubated. We loaded her into the ambulance, and I jumped in the back to help the medic as we made our way to Highland Hospital's trauma center.

There was little we could do for her during the fifteen-to twenty-minute ride to the ER. We wheeled the gurney with the motionless woman on it into the trauma room. Everyone started talking at once, which always happens when a severe trauma comes in. The medic and I lifted the woman off our gurney and onto a hospital bed. As we wheeled the gurney out into the hallway, the blood-stained bed sheet hung halfway off, and the orange seatbelts dangled off the sides. The EKG monitor was still turned on. I took off my gloves and washed my hands. I could still hear the nurses and doctors working to salvage the woman's life.

Medics have to stay at the hospital until they finish their paperwork, and I had to wait for the engine to pick me up. I felt trapped. But when I overheard a social worker telling the nurse she contacted the woman's husband—"He's on his way"—I went cold.

I need to get the fuck out of here before the husband arrives. I didn't want to see him sprinting panicked into the ER as I'd watched other family members do countless times before. I trotted to the door that led to the ambulance outside of the emergency room. I climbed into the back of the ambulance and helped the medics clean up and put their ambulance back together so I could not see anyone outside.

Finally, I heard Engine 6 arrive. I put my head down and gazed at the ground while I walked out to the engine. I climbed into my seat facing backward, watching from where we came, all the way back to quarters. I never saw the husband arrive.

The entire way back to the station, we discussed what to eat for lunch.

Six years after being hired at BFD, I was promoted to apparatus/ operator. Engine 5 had an open driver's spot, which I grabbed. Station 5, on Shattuck and Derby, was my favorite station, and was also the busiest station in the department. It housed an engine, a ladder truck, and an ambulance. I'd also be working for one of the best captains on the fire ground. The front-end truck driver, Drew, was also a good friend of mine and one of the best firefighters we had in our department. I couldn't wait to work with a strong crew who I knew had a passion for this job and worked hard to be good at it. Being on the south side of Berkeley that borders with Oakland, we ran lots of calls and lots of fires.

I quickly gelled with my captain, Cory, and we trusted each other. We both knew the other one was going to make good decisions on the fire ground. He appreciated my high standards. We trained behind the station, and we trained a lot, which was very different from the first two stations I worked at. This station had one of the two trucks so other engine companies, and especially with probationary firefighters, would come and practice raising ladders here. Trucks carried a large cadre of ladders.

After a fire and getting our rigs and everything put back together, we would clean chainsaws and tools we had used during the fire. This happened at all times of the day and night. Great conversations also happened.

A few years into my assignment at Station 5, a handful of us were in the shop, at about 2:00 a.m. after a fire, cleaning tools. We engaged in our usual banter. Drew was cleaning a chainsaw. This meant taking the chain, the bar (the chain spinned around the bar), and other components off the saw, cleaning all the pieces, and putting it back together. I didn't pay close attention to exactly what he was doing, but I watched while he started it and revved it up, making sure it ran okay. Then he started walking toward me. I figured he was going outside. Instead, he came right for me with the engine revved and put the chainsaw blade against my leg. My brain did that slow motion, "Noooo . . ."

Drew hadn't put the chain on, so it was a harmless prank. He and the others in our tool shop burst out laughing. I just keep saying "fuck" over and over, while I waited for my heart rate to come down. Once my brain finally settled down, I burst out laughing, too.

Together, we all watched movies and sporting events, washed our apparatus, and ate. We didn't need to communicate much on calls. We all knew what the other was going to do, and we knew we could count on each other.

When I was at work, Lisa and I got into the routine of talking on the phone at 8:00 p.m. That time seemed to be the greatest chance I had of being in the station.

One night when she called, I went into my room for some privacy, picked up the line, and said, "Hey you, how goes it?"

"It's good, how about you?" Lisa asked. "How has your shift been so far?"

I filled her in on the calls we'd been on, and when I was done, she asked, "Are you going to be able to come home tomorrow?"

"I should. I am low on the mandatory list and the shift is full for tomorrow. What are your plans?"

"Well, that depends on what walks through the front door in the morning."

In the several years of our relationship, Lisa had been saying this to me almost every time we talked the night before I came home. I always assumed she meant how tired I was going to be due to how busy we were going to be at night.

I later figured out she meant something else.

CHAPTER TWELVE

On July 21, 2007, Engine 5 ran calls most of the night. I finally flopped into bed around 4:00 a.m. At 7:00 a.m., I begrudgingly rolled myself out of bed. I started disassembling my bedding when a hard knock came at my door. I opened it and saw Drew with a serious look on his face.

"Con Fire snuffed two firefighters last night."

"What? You are kidding me."

"No, I'm not. It's on the news, and Frank just called me."

"Holy fuck. What happened?"

Matt Burton—the guy whose head I shaved the first week of training—and another guy I knew, Scott, had been killed trying to save two people trapped in a fire. Multiple variables went sideways and because of many small mistakes, they had both burned to death.

Matt and I had gone through fire academy together. Even when we didn't keep in touch, academy mates always shared a kinship. Matt was a great guy. He only wanted to be a firefighter. Matt had gone through all the same crap I'd gone through to get my job—and now his life was over, and his two young kids had lost their dad.

Most days I drove to work, a thought dashed through my head. *I wonder if today is the day.* After Matt and Scott were killed, the thought lingered a little longer.

I worked an overtime shift on Truck Two. Over the PA someone called, "Come and get lunch!"

Plates with giant Philly cheese steak sandwiches plunked down onto the long wooden dining room table. The sound of chairs sliding back and forth on the linoleum filled the dining area. Because of the frequency of the calls at Station 2, sometimes we got one bite, sometimes none, so when food went down on the table, we all acted fast.

While we ate, the dispatch lights and speakers came on, and we all stopped to see who it was for, since the station housed a truck, engine, ambulance, and the battalion chief. The engine and the ambulance were dispatched to an auto vs. pedestrian. Since I was on the truck, I kept eating.

A few minutes later, the alarm went off again. This time, the truck was to respond to the same scene on the UC Berkeley campus. The engine told us over the radio a pedestrian was trapped under a vehicle, and they needed us for extrication.

Fuck. The engine and ambulance are sitting there helpless, waiting for us to extract the person before they could tend to him.

The truck accelerated. Once on campus, our fury boiled at the students who wandered in front of us on the road, slowing us down. The water delivery truck sat motionless in the middle of campus.

The front-end driver and I jumped out of our cabs and began off-loading equipment we needed to raise the delivery truck off the person trapped underneath. We worked furiously to connect air hoses, a regulator, air bags, and an air bottle. The second we raised the water truck high enough, the paramedic belly-crawled under the truck and dragged the man out.

As soon as we saw him, we knew he was dead. Everything stopped as quick as it started. No one moved for a few moments. My driver and I remained kneeling on the asphalt and just looked at each other.

I stood up to stretch and rub my knees. My vision swung to the driver who'd backed up over the now-dead man. This driver, delivering water and going about his day, accidentally killed another human being. His face expressed immeasurable anguish. My heart ached for him. I walked over and gave him a pat him on the shoulder and fumbled for something to say to lessen his pain.

"I'm really sorry." That's all I could come up with. I wanted him to know he was still the same good person he was before this happened.

He stared straight ahead, his shoulders slumped and his hands on his legs. The only movement was his chest heaving as he sobbed.

We cleaned up and put all our equipment back, ready for the next call. As we drove back through the campus, submission replaced urgency. The front-end driver and I drove back to the station on autopilot. No one spoke a word. We patiently waited for the meandering students to get out of our way. We returned to the station and quietly finished our sandwiches.

That afternoon, I wondered if today's accident would make the news. The evening news reported the man we pulled out was a highly esteemed and well-loved professor. A UC Berkeley spokesperson stated the campus community was devastated. This story ended up in the newspaper the next day, too. With each report, I felt a greater pull to say, like a side note to the story, "I'm sorry we couldn't save him."

When events make the news, especially large incidents, first responders are dragged through the event over and over. When a large incident happens, many people ask about it. "Were you there?"

"How bad was it?"

They wanted to know the details. We didn't get to escape our work or the reverberating impact of it.

As usual, the only thing to do was shut down. So, just like every other death I'd witnessed or life I'd failed to save, I put the professor into the box and closed the lid.

In August 2008, Lisa and I sat outside on our patio. We had been together for thirteen years.

"So what do you want for your birthday?" I asked her. "It's coming up in a couple of weeks."

"I want to get married," she said.

"What? You want to get married to me?" I never thought I was someone worthy of marrying, especially to Lisa. She's so smart and responsible. She organized everything surrounding her. Everything had a purpose, or it was gone. She didn't procrastinate and thought everything through. I was a master procrastinator. I had a difficult time throwing things away. We had said we were as good as married, and we would get married if it was legal. But saying that we'd get married when there was no possibility of getting married was easy.

"Ya, of course."

"I knew we were spending the rest of our lives together but getting married is a business agreement." I had always dreamed of being married, of having a partner for life, and I always knew Lisa was the one.

"I still want to marry you for my birthday. We really should do it soon before the government changes their minds and makes it illegal again."

Just a couple of months earlier, California had issued its first same-sex marriage license after California's supreme court overturned the ban on gay marriage. We weren't sure how long it would last. Lisa was right. If we were going to do it, we needed to do it now.

Prior to getting married, I had no idea how deep the connection created between the two of us would feel. Getting married on August 22 at the Martinez courthouse was much more than a piece of paper.

CHAPTER THIRTEEN

It was during my tenure at BFD that I learned to drink alcohol. I'd done the typical drinking in high school and at UC Davis, but once I left the dorms, I never thought about drinking. Lisa didn't drink, so it wasn't part of our lifestyle. But once I settled in at Berkeley Fire and made some friends, I assimilated into a microcosm centered around alcohol. I never even realized it was happening. I went from not having any alcohol in the house to having a liquor cabinet I coveted.

Occasionally, a friend—another firefighter from BFD—and I would meet for breakfast after getting off shift in the morning. A celebratory shot of whiskey or a beer accompanied our eggs, bacon, and coffee, even if we were only celebrating that it was some random Tuesday. When someone got promoted, they footed the bar tab for everyone who showed up at Henry's on Durant after getting off shift. Social events, charity events, and any event revolved around a bar or a brewery, regardless of the time of day. A notable alcohol-fueled story or two always came out of any retirement dinner or evening gathering. It was part of working for any fire or police department.

I became good friends with a guy on my shift, Geissenger, who taught me how to drink Irish whiskey and Jack and Sevens. Geiss was one of the most respected guys in our department. He was exceptionally good at shredding any kind of cockiness or

BS out of someone. He never talked about himself, and he was cool without trying to be. During a rocky time in his marriage, we ended up hanging out together a lot—and all of our times together involved alcohol. We didn't get drunk or overdo it, but alcohol always came along for the ride.

During my gallivanting with Geiss, I grew fond of Irish whiskey and beer.

My shoulder had been bothering me for at least six months, but that didn't stop me from working or regularly playing pickup hockey at Dublin Iceland, about thirty minutes from Berkeley. November 2008, I was on the ice playing one day when a large dude plowed right into me.

My lower right leg folded in half as he drilled me into the ice.

I heard someone yell, "I called 911!!"

I immediately yelled, "Oh man don't do that. Please cancel them!"

A few guys helped me off the ice and to a bench. Before I knew it, an engine crew walked in. I told them I was fine, but they insisted on checking me out. I saw the captain's name tag and realized he was the brother of one of my favorite captains at BFD. When they offered me pain meds, I declined.

"No thank you, I'm fine." I focused on the ambulance. "Can you please cancel them?"

No sooner had I said that then on cue, the paramedics strolled in, including Henry, a guy who wanted to become a firefighter at my department. I knew him well, as he often came by the station for advice on what to do to get hired. All of us at Station 5 liked him.

"Holy crap, hi Henry, fancy meeting you here. I'm sure my leg is broken but it's not an emergency. I don't need an ambulance," I said.

"Well, let me ask, what hospital do you go to?"

"Alta Bates. But seriously, I can get myself there."

I needed to go to the emergency room but not in an ambulance, since I thought it was a weak thing to do. My leg was just broken, I wasn't going to die. I often got frustrated when someone called 911 for something they could easily deal with on their own. Only three ambulances cover the entire city of Berkeley. If all three of them were on a call, regardless of how unnecessary the need for an ambulance was, and another call came in, for example, a baby not breathing, there would be no ambulance in the city to respond to the baby not breathing. An ambulance would be called in from neighboring cities such as Oakland, Albany, or Piedmont. We would get particularly frustrated when these needless calls came in the middle of the night.

"Actually," Henry said, "we have been trying to get back to North Oakland all day. If we take you to Alta Bates, we will back in our own district and not stuck out here. So, you would actually help us out if we took you."

"Okay, only if this is helping you guys out." I stood up to hobble up the stairs, but Henry and his crew insisted on carrying the gurney down to me and then carrying me up the stairs. I argued with them. "I'm fine, I can get up the stairs!" But down came the gurney.

As they wheeled me through the lobby of the ice rink, I wished I could disappear. I didn't want anyone to see me, I was so ashamed. Once they loaded me into the ambulance and tossed my stuff in, I asked Henry's partner, who was in the back with me while Henry drove, if I could make a phone call. She nodded as she took my left arm to start an IV.

"Do you want any pain meds?" she asked.

"No, thank you. I'm fine." I dialed Lisa with my right hand, but the call went straight to voicemail. I was hoping to catch her before she left the office to see if she could catch a ride to pick up my car at Iceland.

"Shit, she isn't answering."

The medic started an IV. By now thirty minutes had passed since I'd hit the ice and my leg began to hurt.

The medic asked me, "Are you sure you don't want any pain meds?"

This time I said, "Yeah, why not? It's starting to hurt."

She administered morphine, and the pain eased up. Then, like a warm wave, the nausea hit.

"Oh man, I don't feel so good. I think I am going to barf." She casually handed me a basin.

I tried Lisa one more time and this time she answered. "Hey, are you all right? I was in a meeting and saw you call a few times."

"I broke my leg at pickup in Dublin and I'm in a stupid ambulance on my way to Alta Bates."

Lisa went into fixer mode. "Okay," she said calmly, "I'll be on my way in just a few minutes."

I was already dreading having to ask someone to help me get my car back home from the ice rink. Then I remembered when I had pulled into the ice rink parking lot, Tenacious D's "Fuck Her Gently" had been playing. Loud.

Oh crap, whoever starts up my car will hear that song blasting out.

Twenty minutes later, we pulled onto the emergency room ramp, something I had done hundreds of times myself, only this time my view looked out the back windows instead of the front. A nurse I knew met us at the ER doors. A handful of my coworkers happened to be in the ER, dropping off patients. They rolled the gurney into a room and went through all the motions they normally went through.

It was so strange to be on the other side. Several of my coworkers, a couple of nurses, and the doctor came in. I knew everyone in the room. They gathered around me to witness the removal of my hockey shin guard in anticipation of some horrible deformity since I was so sure it was broken. The suspense of everyone standing and looking over my leg deserved a drum roll. The doctor carefully lifted the shin guard and exposed my bare leg. And there was . . . nothing. Not a bump, not a bruise, no swelling, nothing. My leg looked completely normal. Everyone sighed, a few of them rolled their eyes, and my room emptied.

"I swear it's broken!" I said. "I even feel crepitus in there!"

I felt like an idiot. I had just been outed as a fucking pussy. *I should have never come here. I should have just gone home and sucked it up.* I was already embarrassed to go to the ER in an ambulance. I complained relentlessly when people called for an ambulance ride to the hospital when they didn't need one. I had just become everything I hated—the patient who couldn't take care of herself or handle a little bit of pain. And now I had no outward evidence of my pain. I knew what I would think of myself if I were them.

A chatty technician rolled my bed into X-ray. I was not talkative, but her kindness and cheerful mood didn't allow me to be a complete jerk. She covered my reproductive organs with a lead apron and moved my leg around—a lot.

After taking the X-rays she said, "Oh yeah, you broke your leg."

I felt some redemption, but the X-ray tech couldn't fix what everyone had seen. Or rather hadn't seen. I was wheeled back into my room where a nurse entered to offer me more pain meds.

"I know they moved your leg around in X-ray. It's gotta be hurting. Are you sure you don't want anything for the pain?"

I said, "Naw. I'm fine. Thank you, though."

My leg throbbed with pain but there was no way I was going to take more pain meds for most likely a puny fracture that did not even cause a bruise.

About ten minutes later, one of my firefighter pals who had witnessed the dramatic unveiling of my perfectly fine-looking leg came in and said, "Have you seen the X-ray?"

"No, but the X-ray tech said it's broken."

"Here, let me show you," he said. He unlocked my hospital bed and rolled me out of my room and over to the X-Ray light box. "You did yourself a good one," he said.

My fibula looked like a splintered tree branch snapped in two. No wonder it hurt.

My coworker rolled me back into my room and a nurse followed.

"Would you like some pain meds now?" she asked.

"Yes, please," I said, sheepishly.

That evening, they sent me home with my leg in a soft cast. I laid on the couch with my leg propped up, holding a large bowl to throw up in. It was late, and Lisa sat with me.

"Well," I said, "I might as well get my shoulder fixed now. I'll be off work anyway."

"That's a good idea. Do you need anything?"

"I'm fine. You can go to bed."

I didn't want to burden Lisa any more than I already had. I would have loved for her to stay with me, but I knew I could handle whatever I needed to by myself.

"I feel so bad for you. I wish there was something I could do."

"I'm all right. You've already done a lot." The pain in my leg had become intense, and I had a difficult time focusing on anything else.

"I'll sit with you for a bit."

We both stayed quiet as she sat with me for a while longer and then went to bed.

I got a referral to an orthopedist for the following day who informed me I wouldn't be able to go back to work for three to four months. The doctor put my leg in a permanent cast and gave me crutches.

When I got home, I made the appointment to see the shoulder surgeon. The surgeon expressed some hesitation in doing the surgery so close to getting out of my cast.

"Are you sure you don't want to wait a week? That really seems like a lot."

In my most reassuring voice I said, "Oh geez, I'll be totally fine."

Since I broke my leg while off duty and I hadn't filed a workers' comp claim for my shoulder, I would have to use my sick leave and vacation time. I filed for FMLSA, the Family Medical Leave Act, which legally allowed me to be off work for twelve weeks—and the city could not fire me.

I had injured my shoulder on the job, but I and everyone knew the workers' compensation system was a disaster. Workers' comp would immediately deny my claim, and I wouldn't be able to get an MRI or surgery until workers' comp accepted my claim. I knew if I went that route, it would involve hiring a lawyer and everything would be dragged out. So I had ignored my shoulder as best I could until now. At least this way, I had some control over my care.

My first time on crutches made me realize I never wanted to use crutches again. Trying to get something from a room in the house to my chair in the living room was a Herculean effort. I would go into my home gym to work out, only to realize I needed both legs to carry the weights over to the bench I needed to sit on. I also needed to keep my leg elevated or my toes would turn a deep shade of blue. Driving was out of the question, since my right leg was broken.

I quickly found out, however, that beers fit perfectly in my shorts pocket. Almost every day in the late afternoon, I'd crutch my way to the refrigerator, put a beer in my right pocket and a bottle opener in my left pocket. Then I'd crutch back to my recliner, elevate my leg, and drink my beer. Repeat.

Lisa and I struggled during this time. She watched as I did everything I could to take care of myself and not ask for help while throwing my resentfulness all over the house. I was pathetic and felt sorry for myself. Lisa is not a particularly nurturing person; she comes from a family of people who never complained, and her parents always expected her to suck it up. I found her frustration with me confusing.

One day, as I sat in my recliner with my leg elevated, I asked Lisa, "Are you mad at me?"

She frowned and said, "Yes, I'm mad at you! You play hockey and do everything else like you're twelve years old and think there won't be any consequences. You're an adult and you have responsibilities!"

A quiet pause hung in the room. I didn't know how to reply.

I sighed and said, "I'm sorry. If you don't want to help me, then I'll find someone else. I'll go stay with a friend until I don't need any help." I hoped Lisa would tell me how much she loved me and of course she'd take care of me. Instead, I got an angry lecture.

With her hands on her hips she said, "That's not the point. You have responsibilities."

I stared at the wall and said, "I'm sorry."

I always said sorry for everything, even if I had nothing to do with something going wrong. I felt my existence caused problems in other's lives. A part of me ached to be nurtured and cared for. But the risk was too great, since I'd experienced the cost of reaching out and being rejected.

The only person who had unconditionally loved me was

my grandma, who'd died when I was ten. I hadn't gone to her funeral, but my dad, Barbara, and I had visited her gravesite one day not long after her passing. Seeing her headstone made her death real, and my chest began to fill with grief.

I reached for my dad and put my arms around his waist, wanting him to wrap me in comfort. He had patted me on the back and pulled my arms off of him.

Now, as then, I committed to not asking for help. I could do this on my own.

The aftermath of shoulder surgery sucked even more than being on crutches. The doctor and a few nurses warned me to take pain meds before the nerve block wore off, but I was so afraid of my arm being forever dead that I refused to take anything. I wanted to know the moment my arm regained feeling.

But the warning was for good reason, because as soon as that arm woke up, a pain hit like none I'd ever felt before. They also warned me to take stool softeners.

I said to myself, *That's nice, lady, I don't need stool softeners.* I had only known old people to use stool softeners. But it didn't take long before the pain meds completely blocked me up. After lots and lots of water, and lots of stool softeners, my butt gave birth to a ten-pound pineapple.

After a week of pain meds plugging me up, I thought there had to be a better way. The pain med bottles stated, "Do Not Drink Alcohol with this medication. It might intensify the effect."

Perfect! I thought. *An intensified effect is exactly what I need.*

I got up the next morning, walked to the kitchen, and took one pain pill instead of two; then I opened my liquor cabinet, took out a bottle of Jameson, took a large swig off the bottle and put it back on the shelf.

A handful of minutes later, my shoulder pain melted away as did the tension that had built up inside my entire body. I felt better than I had in a week and taking half the amount of opioids also meant I wouldn't be so miserably constipated.

I knew I would never get addicted to pain medication because I didn't like the side effects. Drinking Jameson out of the bottle in the morning, however, proved to be very addictive. It gave me something to look forward to.

Soon, my morning Jameson turned into afternoon Jameson, midafternoon Sierra Nevada, and evening Jack & Seven. I had nowhere to go and nothing to do, so what the hell? I couldn't even brush my teeth or wash my hair with this arm, so how in the fuck would it ever be possible to lift a ladder or chainsaw over my head again?

Two weeks after surgery, I started physical therapy. The doctor wanted to get my shoulder moving as soon as possible but only passive movement by the physical therapist.

At my first appointment, the first question the physical therapist asked was, "How much pain are you in?"

"Ahhh, quite a bit," I said.

"When was the last time you took any pain meds?"

"A couple of days ago."

"Why aren't you taking your pain meds?"

"I dunno. I don't feel like I should still need them after two weeks."

The physical therapist said, "That's the most ridiculous thought I have heard. If you are in pain, you need to take the pain medication."

I looked at him as if he spoke a foreign language. What he said made sense—for everyone else. I was not everyone else. I could handle pain. I wouldn't be weak and take pain meds for longer than necessary. Between the increased pain after physical therapy and his "permission" to still take pain meds, I started them again.

For the next few months, I sat pissed off in my recliner. Lisa left the house at 6:00 a.m. for work and came home around 5:00 p.m. I was moody, irritated, and threw a grand pity party for myself. The thought I could lose my job if my recovery took too long or my shoulder was so badly damaged that I could never go back scared me shitless. I was sure losing my job would be the very worst thing that could happen to me. I stewed over this fear, a quiet panic brewing inside of me.

Lisa would say to me, "You know your shoulder and leg are going to get better?"

"It sure doesn't feel like it."

I ended up being off work for nine months. Nine months of sitting in a chair with my leg up, my shoulder in a sling, going to physical therapy, feeling alone, and missing my job.

I managed to whittle down my drinking to just a couple every day as I got closer to being able to start work again. I knew that to get back to work, not only did I have to make sure my leg and shoulder felt good, I also had to get back into shape. And I couldn't wait to get back to Station 5 and my peers, to have meals together, hear the tones go off, smell the smoke in the engine, and feel like I belonged. I worked my ass off to get my fitness back.

When the day finally approached, I received an email congratulating a coworker for getting promoted to apparatus/operator. The email stated he would be the engine driver on Engine 5, my spot. It also added I would be moved to the apparatus/operator spot at Station 3. I stared at my computer screen for almost a minute. Several cuss words flew out of my mouth.

I didn't even know what to say. The floor had been ripped out from underneath me. I needed the challenge of Station 5. I felt valued as a human being when working at a busy, hard-driving station. Station 5 ran more calls, and those calls were of a much greater variety than 3. Station 5's district served a more diverse socio-economic community and responded to more fires. Station 3 could be slow during the day but it was always busy at night because of its location near UC Berkeley—and most of the calls were all the same, dealing with drunk college students.

I had been so happy at Station 5. I had been looking forward to getting back to the type of calls in that district, the station itself, and working with Drew and the other guys assigned to that station. Being moved to Station 3 felt like being kicked off the island.

CHAPTER FOURTEEN

Fire Station 3, on Russell and College Avenue, covered the southeast corner of Berkeley. Station 3's district included almost all the UC Berkeley fraternities, sororities, several large co-ops, which were large buildings housing thirty-plus students who partied and trashed their own housing regularly, and about half of the student dorms. The district included five thousand-plus-square-foot homes. Many of these large houses were built with the garage on the first floor and the rest of the house built downward, against the hill. The district included large two-to-three-story Victorians that had been chopped up into tiny apartments/boarding rooms without building permits. From a fire perspective, they're basically death traps. The district also had, as Berkeley called them, "traffic-calming devices" so streets were effectively blocked, making it more difficult to get from point A to point B.

This district also covered Telegraph Ave and People's Park. During the day, Telegraph Ave was vibrant with peace, love, and food. At night, Telegraph Ave was all about booze, fights, and lighting trash cans on fire.

People's Park, just a block off Telegraph, was a soup of the homeless suffering from mental health issues. We ran mostly medical calls there although, occasionally, something interesting would happen. For instance, one time we responded to multiple people engaged in a sword fight. Just when we thought we'd seen it all in Berkeley.

During the UC Berkeley school year, Engine 3 ran calls all night—mostly college students who'd done something to hurt themselves or others because of their drunkenness, and false fire alarms relentlessly set off by accident or on purpose. We had to respond to each alarm as if there was an actual fire. That meant putting our fifty pounds of gear on and walking through a large and usually filthy fraternity house or marching up six flights of stairs in a dorm at 2:00 a.m. only to find a resident taking an extra-long hot shower and the steam had set off the smoke detector, and in turn, the fire alarm. It wasn't a rarity to have the fire alarm pulled at the same dorm three times in one night.

I was, at least, driving for a captain I had a great deal of respect for. It was great to be working again for someone who had their shit together. But she was one of the few bright spots in my new job.

Every year at the beginning of wildland season—what the public called fire season, when we entered the warm, dry months—Engine 3, along with several other engines, took part in an afternoon wildland drill in the Berkeley hills. These drills included developing hundreds of feet of hose lays, using tools such as shovels to develop fire lines and clear brush, and shuttling water to the engine that pumped to the hose lines.

At one of these drills, we used our entire five-hundred-gallon water tank. When the drill ended and we left Tilden Park, the closest most accessible hydrant was being used by another engine who'd participated in the same drill. We decided not to wait for that hydrant and to head back to our district instead, as having an engine without water in our district was better than having no engine at all. We planned to fill up at the hydrant in front of our station.

When we arrived at the station, I backed the engine into the apparatus floor, also known as the garage, and shut the engine off. The quiet was soothing. We changed out of our wildland gear and into workout clothes. I cleaned the tools we used and cleaned up the engine full of mud and dried grass plus a healthy layer of dust inside and out. The captain went into her office and began paperwork. One of the guys started cooking dinner for the station.

We got lucky to have a slow night. Dinner was on time, then we cleaned up, watched TV, and went to bed. It ended up being one of the very rare nights we slept all night since I'd been at Berkeley.

The next morning, at around 7:30 a.m., Todd, my A/O relief, walked into the station with his normal good mood and cheery demeanor. I told Todd the status of the engine.

"Everything's good. We did a wildland drill yesterday, but everything has been cleaned and put back. And holy crap, we slept all night!"

I came home in an unusually good mood.

Sixteen hours after waking up at work, as I lay in bed trying to fall asleep, out of nowhere I suddenly remembered, *I fucking forgot to fill the engine water tank. I went the whole evening and into the night on an empty water tank. I turned the engine over without water in the tank!*

My mind raced. Should I call and wake up Todd and tell him? What do I do? I'm sure he caught it on the daily morning checkout. If we ran any calls during the night, I would have noticed the red lights on the pump panel indicating the tank was empty. But we fucking slept all night. Fuck!

I could have been responsible for someone's death or their house not being saved. One mistake could have resulted in a disaster. If someone had turned the engine over to me like that, and especially if it had been someone I didn't like, I would have thrown a tantrum and let everyone know how enormously the person had fucked up. If it had been someone I liked, though, I would have covered for them.

I didn't sleep the rest of the night, going over and over in my mind that I could have been responsible for something catastrophic.

The next morning, as soon as I thought I wouldn't be waking up the entire station, I called Todd.

He said, "It's all okay. I saw it right away when I was doing my checkout."

"I am so so sorry, Todd." I couldn't stop apologizing.

He said, "Yeah, that could have been bad, but it's okay. Shit happens."

The next shift I told my captain how I had blown it and forgot to fill the tank.

She said, "Holy shit, are you kidding me? Thank God we didn't go on a fire." And then went about her day.

No one yelled at me. No one talked behind my back. My captain and Todd allowed for mistakes, which helped me realize we're all human. But I had much greater expectations of myself. I expected perfection and to never make a mistake like that. This error did not go into the box. I let this one beat the crap out of me for a while.

Almost a year later, in May 2011, my skate caught a small divot in the ice while I was playing ice hockey, I fell backward, and I felt my lower leg—not the one I had broken before—snap.

As I laid in a small heap on the ice, everyone came over to help.

"What happened? Are you all right?" My hockey mates hovered over me.

"I am fine, just give me a minute."

Liz, one of my teammates, yelled, "Call an ambulance!"

I sternly told her, "No! Do not call an ambulance! I just broke my leg! I'm fine!"

My friends/teammates helped me up and to the bench. It was the beginning of the game. I had carpooled with a friend, Evelyn, and I didn't want her to miss the game.

She climbed over the boards and said, "Let me go change, and I will take you to the ER." I replied, "No way, finish the game. It doesn't hurt that bad. I'm fine."

"Are you sure? You broke your leg."

"I'm positive. I'll totally be fine. The game just started. Totally go play it."

"Okay. But if you change your mind, let me know."

"I will," I said, knowing I wouldn't.

I sat on the end of the ice side team bench for a few minutes when a woman I knew from league, Linda, who sat at the bar above the ice, came down and asked, "Do you need any help getting into the locker room?"

"That'd be great," I said, thankful she came down. I didn't want to sit for an hour on the bench where the air was freezing cold. Plus, I wanted to change, and I needed to call Lisa.

She put her arms out in front of her and said, "Do you want me to just carry you?" She was totally serious.

Linda was tall and strong; she was fully capable of carrying me. But inside my head I laughed and thought about what a sight it would be. I would forever be known for Linda carrying me into the locker room.

"Thank you, but no. Can you just help me walk?"

She helped me hobble down the hallway. Inside, I sat down on the locker room bench. This room was usually full of people, chatter, laughter, and shenanigans while we changed into or out of our hockey gear. The quiet emptiness in the room, with the entire team's hockey bags strewn about, immediately brought back the feeling of being left behind. My teammates were all together, and I sat in here alone. I lay my broken leg up onto the bench. The call home I needed to make filled me with dread.

After staring at my phone for a full minute, I took a deep breath and dialed.

Before I could say anything, Lisa said, "Did you break your leg again?"

She knew I was only about ten minutes into my game, so she'd already figured out something was wrong.

I hung my head, "Um . . . yeah."

"Goddammit!"

"I'm sorry! I wasn't doing anything crazy, I promise! Can you grab my crutches and bring them to the ER? Evelyn will drive me and my car to Alta Bates Hospital."

Lisa was pissed. I was pissed. I couldn't believe I'd done this again.

I did the best I could at getting out of my hockey gear and into my clothes. I waited for about an hour in the locker room until the game ended. By then, my leg was throbbing.

Finally, my team came back, filling the room with the familiar, comforting banter and noise. Evelyn dressed quickly and then some of my friends from the other team came in and asked if I was okay.

One of them looked at me and asked, "How are we going to get you out to the car?"

"Find an office chair with wheels on it, and you can just roll me out," I said.

While waiting for a chair, Linda produced a bottle of Jameson and handed it to me. Everyone seemed to know Jameson was my favorite. I drew a couple of big swigs out of the bottle to help with the pain. I had also sent Evelyn, who carpooled with me to the game, to get my car and bring it to the entrance of the ice rink. Evelyn was wonderful and brilliant, but she was the worst person I could have sent to find the car because she can be a little dingy. She walked back in just as I was sliding into a chair with wheels on it and announced, "Someone stole your car."

"Are you serious? Wait, are you sure?"

"I looked everywhere! It's not out there."

"It's gotta be out there."

I told her again exactly where I'd parked it. She headed back out to the parking lot. Ten minutes later, she came back and told me she'd found it and had pulled it up front.

I smiled and said, "I knew you could do it!" and we both laughed.

Sitting on my chair with wheels, Jameson onboard, my friends from the team wheeled me out to my car that wasn't stolen. My hockey teammates used this opportunity to make many jokes at my expense. I stood on one leg and gingerly lowered myself in the passenger seat. Evelyn climbed into the driver's seat and off we went to Alta Bates emergency room.

And so it began. Again. It would be another three to four months before I could go back to work. I had learned many tricks from the last time I spent weeks on crutches, such as how beers fit perfectly in my pockets. Lisa grabbed me the same five-gallon bucket for me to sit on in the shower and the same sturdy pillows out of the closet to elevate my leg.

I was grateful I could drive since this time I'd broken my left leg. But I didn't go out much because if I did not elevate my leg for a while, my toes would turn a dark shade of blue and purple. I again threw myself another pity party, but this one didn't last as long because I'd been through this before. I knew I'd get better, and my job would be waiting for me.

But just like last time, Lisa was mad at me.

After two weeks, Lisa's anger dissipated.

"How are you?" she asked me one day.

I answered honestly, "I am so uncomfortable, it hurts to sit still or to move around."

Instead of saying, "Well you should be more careful" like she had before, this time she said, "I'm so sorry. Is there anything I can do for you? I wish I could make your leg better."

"Thank you," I said. "I appreciate that. I'm gonna have a few cocktails and watch *Xena: Warrior Princess.*"

Lisa chuckled and said "So, has it come to this?"

"Yes, it has come to this." I replied.

"You get one more leg break while playing hockey and then you are done."

"I totally agree with you. From now on instead of playing to win, I will play to be able to drive myself home and go to work the next day."

After six weeks of being in a cast, the doctor finally cut it off. I performed all the physical therapy and strengthened my leg and everything else that had atrophied. I went back to work just in time for UC Berkeley's fall classes to start and the Station 3 shit show to begin.

Once I returned to work, my new thing was to drink a Jameson or two the evening right before my shift. I'd tell Lisa, "This is my 'if I don't come back' drink."

Soon enough I started having a drink or two my first night home from work, too. One evening, I sat in front of the TV, having just sucked down three drinks and feeling pretty good. Across the TV screen, interrupting the hockey game I was watching, came a breaking news report. A large apartment-over-commercial building fire in Berkeley had quickly risen to three alarms.

My eyes fixated on the TV footage. *Holy shit! That is one big fire.* The building was in my district, and I had been in that building several times. I knew the maze of hallways and apartments inside.

My phone blew up with texts from a department all-call. They wanted everyone who was able to come into work. *But I am buzzed from having a few drinks. Son of a bitch, I won't be going anywhere.*

The rest of the evening, I pretended not to give a shit I was missing a once-in-a-career fire. But I could not stop watching news footage, the one everyone else would be at and tell stories about and build camaraderie over. I stewed at what I was missing all because I'd had a few drinks.

The last news footage we saw before I went to bed showed the large building with fire blowing out of every window and hundreds of feet of hose tangled on the ground, looking like a giant bowl of pasta. Anger roiled and boiled inside of me, but I didn't say anything. It was my own fault.

Instead of talking to Lisa about this, I said, "Fuck me. Look at all that hose I am going to have to clean up when I go into work tomorrow. What a mess."

My friends and family, bursting with excitement, would later ask me, "Where you at that huge fire?"

I had to respond, "No, I wasn't there."

The disappointment on their faces deepened my disappointment and sense of failure. This was a symptom of basing my value and worth in life on the job.

CHAPTER FIFTEEN

At the end of January 2012, the fire chief and my battalion chief came to my station and asked the crew to assemble at the dining room table.

The fire chief said to the group, "I am proud to announce Christy has been promoted to the rank of captain." She shook my hand and handed me a captain's badge. "Your assignment will remain at Station 3, and a badge-pinning ceremony will be held at a date to be determined."

I admired my new captain's badge and rolled it around in my hand. "Thank you for this." After the chiefs left, the guys patted me on the back, congratulated me, and explained how much ice cream I owed them. When someone was promoted or on TV, they had to buy the station or the department ice cream. I walked back to my room and took my uniform shirt off. I removed my apparatus/operators badge and put my captain's badge on my uniform.

Receiving the badge gave me a great sense of relief and excitement. Being a captain gave me control over what was important to me. I could make sure my crews were taken care of and that we treated every person with respect that we came in contact with. When I saw something happening that I believed was wrong, I could stop it. I'd been hoping for this for a long time. I was content.

After I made captain, every night when I crawled into bed at work, I'd lay there and think of a handful of scenarios that could occur in my district in the middle of the night. I developed plans with different options and variables. A large two-story house with fire on the first floor and people trapped on the second. Where would I enter with my hose line? Should I put the fire out first or go through the second-story window and start rescuing people? How big was the fire and exactly where was it on the first floor? If I started rescuing people from the second floor and didn't put out the fire, would the fire spread to the second floor before I could get everyone out? What if my second-due engine and the truck were on a call and it would be too many minutes until the next engine came? The second-due engine was the engine that arrived on scene second. The second due engine usually connected the first engine to a water supply. What if the ambulance from our station was on a call so it was just the three of us? What if the ambulance responded with us, and there were two new guys on it who had never been into a structure fire before? What if? What if?

All those thoughts were for just one type of house. When I'd run through every possible scenario for one type, I'd moved onto the next. When I got ripped from a deep sleep to go to a three-story house on fire with people trapped, I'd hopefully already have a plan in my head I could roll out before I shook loose the cobwebs, and I was fully awake, thinking clearly.

On my third shift as a captain, the driver assigned to me was a guy who'd been in the department for years and was filling in for a single shift. We were in the engine, just about to pull out of the station.

He said to me, "If you get me killed, I am going to come back as a ghost and slit your throat. All right?"

The serious look on his face and his tone of voice indicated he was serious.

I put the onus back on him. "Well, then don't do anything that you don't feel safe doing."

He glanced at me and said, "People here at the department will work with you, but none of us want to go have a beer with you."

I took that as a compliment. "I'm here to do a job and do it well. Making friends is great but that's not why I'm here."

An unspoken rule in the fire service was we would die for one another. It had always been the case my crew came first, but now that I worked in a leadership role, this held true even more. I would give my life for this guy in an instant, even though he'd basically just threatened to kill me. I wanted people to like me—but I needed them to think I was a good firefighter.

During the first six months of being a captain, some turnover of drivers occurred due to retirements and administration moving people around to balance the shifts. Finally, the department assigned Engine 3 a permanent driver—Bobby Law. Bobby Law was the size of two of me—six-foot-five and solid. He was also incredibly smart. We clicked. Our dynamic was like the work version of what I had with Lisa. What one of us was not good at, the other one was. This was the relationship I had always dreamed of having in the fire service. We were loyal and had each other's backs one hundred percent.

On October 3, ten months after my promotion, the light and speaker activated in the middle of the night. The familiar mechanized voice said, "Engine 3," followed by several *blips, bleeps*, and *bloops*. "Sending a full assignment for a propane tank on fire in the rear of "XXXX" address."

A full assignment designated a standard response of one truck, four engines, an ambulance, and a battalion chief. The location was around the corner, and dispatch let us know it was a small fire. It would be a quick and easy one.

My brain struggled to wake up as I made my way to the apparatus bay. Being the first one there, I hit the button to the metal roll-up door. Footsteps plodded down the stairs and the familiar swoosh of the pneumatic door to the engine opened once, then again, and again. We all quietly but quickly put on our gear. I climbed up the steps into the captain's seat, hit the "responding" box on the computer, and put my headset on.

"I'll find the propane tank and you pull the line," I said to my firefighter. "It sounds like it's in the backyard. You know the deal. You cool the tank, and I will shut off the valve." I knew we'd be back in bed in no time.

We turned the corner and holy fuck—the entire second floor of a 3,500-square-foot, two-story house was on fire. Now I was awake . . . wide awake.

On the radio, dispatch said, "Be advised PD is on scene and says it is fully engulfed and there may be people trapped inside."

We came to a lurching stop in front of the house. From the peaceful quiet inside the cab, I gave my condition report on the radio. When I opened the door, noise made the air thick. My firefighter and I flaked out the hose line and headed for the front door. I called to Bobby Law for water and watched the pressurized water snake through the hose toward us and to the nozzle.

My firefighter and I made entry into the house to search for any possible victims still inside. My firefighter directed the hose stream on and up the stairs to hold the fire from coming back down into the first floor of the house. This bought us time so I could continue searching. While in the back of the house, my radio blasted out.

"Get out of the house," Bobby's voice shouted. "We lost our supply." This meant the hose feeding the engine with water came off the hydrant.

"Get out of there!" the battalion chief yelled from outside.

I had my firefighter stay in the hallway by the door with the still-pressurized hose line while I finished searching the house; then we exited the building together. While the conditions were still tenable, I wasn't leaving anyone behind.

The water supply line was reconnected to the hydrant, but we couldn't go back in. The fire had grown so large we could not get inside anymore. We had to attack the fire from the outside.

About forty minutes later, after we'd put the fire out, the real work began—overhaul. This involved opening walls, ceilings, or any other voids to look for fire extension. Firefighters recovered any property that was salvageable and wetted down everything and anything still burning or smoldering. Incident Command sent me and my firefighter to the roof to cut much of it away and to wet down what was left.

Once we were done, I climbed down a ladder off the roof and hobbled out into the street. *Holy fuck, my knee hurts.* I had torn my meniscus while at work about two months prior. I never filed a workers' compensation claim because of the poor quality of their treatment options and then the long wait to get medical care. I used my regular orthopedic doctor and was scheduled to have surgery right after my forty-eight-hour shift ended. The pain had been manageable, but that night it screamed, *Get off me!*

I still had twenty-eight hours before my shift ended. I sucked it up while counting down the minutes until I could go home. I'd used all my sick leave for my broken leg and shoulder surgery, so I was trying to build up as much as I could for what I would need after this knee surgery.

Finally, my shift ended. I drove home and took a shower. Then Lisa and I headed to the surgery center. My surgeon cut out the torn part of my meniscus and the next day my knee felt better already, though it would be a couple of months before I'd be able to walk without a limp.

A badge-pinning ceremony was a big deal among firefighters. Everyone dressed in their Class A formal uniforms, there were speeches and a reception afterward. Several members of the city government attended, along with many people from the department and the friends and families of those who were being pinned. At most departments, firefighters chose who would pin them. I chose my wife.

The big day arrived, and I put on my fancy Class A formal uniform, and Lisa, my brother, and I drove into Berkeley, to the Berkeley Repertory Theater. The ceremony started with a speech from the chief.

My knee was still healing. I could walk but with a limp. Stairs were difficult. When my name was called, I gingerly walked to the five-step staircase that led to the stage.

There was no railing to hold onto, so Captain Smith, who was part of the honor guard, gave me his arm to lean on to get up the stairs. I felt like a fucking joke. I believed everyone in the audience, especially the spouses, was thinking, *Typical female. Needs help to get up the stairs.*

In just five short weeks, I'd be getting surgery on my other knee. When my surgeon and I had discussed this possibility, he'd told me, "You have firefighter's knees. It's from carrying heavy weight up and down stairs. I see so many firefighters with knees like yours."

I had never thought of how long my knees would last in this job. All I cared about was getting healed up and back to work. Being laid up and missing work was hard. Pain was easy.

CHAPTER SIXTEEN

September 10, 2013, at about 1:00 a.m., Station 3 was asleep. The overhead red light gently lit up, and the lady with the electronic voice calmly said, "Engine 3" followed by a brief pause. During this pause, my nervous system began to awaken, but my brain remained asleep. I knew I was going on a call, but I had no idea what I'd be responding to. It could be something as innocuous as the usual drunk college student or as significant as a tremendous structure fire with people trapped. The sounds that followed the announcement over the system would decide how much my heart woke up.

The brief pause was followed by several *blip bloop beep* noises. Each blip called for a different piece of equipment. Two blips meant an engine and ambulance or an engine and a truck required. Several blips equaled several pieces of equipment, which was what sputtered out that night. We were responding to something significant. After the blips came an announcement of what the call was for, the address, and the units due.

In a nanosecond, my heart started—first cool and steady, then thumping like Animal from the Muppets was playing the drums in my chest. With that adrenaline dump, the heart woke up much faster than the brain.

"Sending a full assignment to 2025 Oregon Street," the dispatcher announced. "Heavy flames coming from the third story of an apartment building." Then she rattled off all the apparatus due.

2025 Oregon Street was in my district, so we'd be first on scene. I'd decide what door to go through and what hose line to bring in or whether to even take a hose line in if someone was trapped. Countless other decisions had to be made. For example, if the risk of going through the front door seemed too great, should we wait for the second-due engine or the truck company to cut a hole in the roof? These decisions had to be made with a snapshot of incomplete information. It took some skill, but mostly experience and a solid gut check.

As I hurriedly shoved myself into my turnouts, I urged my brain to wake up and clear out the cobwebs of sleep. My crew and I climbed into the engine rubbing our eyes while our hearts pounded inside our chests and our brains strained to figure out what the hell was going on.

As we pulled out of the station, we made a plan. But just as we turned the corner, Engine 5 made a size-up report on the radio. They'd arrived on scene before us.

What? How in the fuck did Engine 5 beat us on scene? We were much closer, and we'd gotten out of the station fast. I couldn't fucking believe this, and I knew I'd never hear the end of this. I got beat into my district.

Later I would learn Engine 5 had just cleared a fire alarm. So not only were they already out, but they were already dressed for a fire.

Now that we were the second engine on scene, we had to shift gears. We'd already driven past the hydrant that the second arriving engine typically connects a large hose to, so we came to a stop and my driver and firefighter hopped out and pulled the end of the heavy five-inch supply hose over their shoulders and dragged it two hundred feet, all the way down the block, back to the hydrant. I walked to the front of the building. Huge flames barreled out of an enormous, round, front window of the penthouse in a three-story apartment building.

While my crew dragged hose, I found Fred, the first-in captain, and asked, "Hey, what do you need?"

He replied, "Two hose packs to the third floor!"

I climbed onto the engine tailboard, pulled on the hose pack loops that sat way above my head, dropped each pack on a shoulder, and took off through the front door. The lobby and the stairwell showed no evidence that the top of the building raged with fire. The air was clear and the stairway was well lit.

The hose line was completed, and the flames were knocked down. Engine 5 and Truck 5 gave the "all clear" on the radio, meaning the primary search had been completed and no victims were found inside. My crew finished completing the supply line connections, and I approached the battalion chief/incident commander for our next assignment.

"The neighbors keep saying there is someone still inside there," he said, almost rolling his eyes. "I doubt it but will you and your crew go inside and look for him? Just make sure he's not in there. Engine 5 and Truck 5 are coming out of the building for new air bottles. I want you to replace them and become Division 3."

That meant my assignment was to supervise the crews and operations on the third floor, where the fire had just been put out. I nodded, gathered my crew, and headed up to the third floor.

The apartment was a modest penthouse. As I made it to the top of the stairs, Truck 5 and Engine 5's crews were amassed in the doorway. Confusion swirled and quite a bit of "interaction" took place before we got them outside and were able to go inside.

The front door led into a hallway that connected the large living room with the rest of the penthouse. The living room was empty, except for the metal coil skeleton of a bed mattress. Fire had consumed everything, turning the room into a blackened shell. The heat of the fire took out the enormous oval window. The hole looked surreal.

I headed to the right and searched the rooms off the hallway, looking for the possibly missing person. The rooms to the right of the front door remained undamaged. Only gray soot brushed the ceiling from smoke. I took a quick look in the kitchen at the far end of the hallway. The kitchen had a tiny bit of soot on the ceiling but otherwise appeared free of any fire damage.

The incident commander assigned Engine 2 to Division 3, and they started overhaul with my crew, opening walls and ceilings to make sure the fire wasn't still burning in places we could not see. I moved to the living room to assess what needed to be done. I stared at a giant hole that had been a front window. It looked just like the "Hey Koolaid" man had just run through the wall. I stood on a mattress in the corner and found the blackened coils still had their bounce.

Just then, my peripheral vision caught rapid movements from the hallway. My head swung to face it, and ten feet in front of me, two firefighters struggled to carry a completely limp and ashen person.

My world instantly flipped and moved in slow motion. I felt as if I were alone in the middle of a scorching desert that stretched for thousands of miles. Two seconds felt like an hour. I'd just made one of the biggest fuckups of my life.

I watched them carry the man by his arms and legs down the hallway, down the stairs, and out of sight. It took only seconds, as the crew moved awkwardly but swiftly—but to me it was like watching a horror film shot in slow motion.

The crew of Engine 2 had finally found him, and they weren't even looking for him. As they pulled ceiling, one of them saw something under the kitchen table, against the wall, that didn't appear quite right. It was him; the person I never finished searching for.

After we finished salvage and mop up, we returned to the station and went about after-fire routines. We helped Bobby clean up the engine equipment. We took showers as we always did, blowing black snot out of our noses. We poured ourselves cups of coffee, and we all filtered in and out of the kitchen, searching for something to eat. I shoved my misery deep down into the box where no one could see it. I wrote my reports, put my dirty, smoky, carcinogenic turnouts into the wash, and got ready to go home.

But I couldn't keep the limp, gray, and ashen person inside my misery box this time. He kept spilling out over the sides. I didn't know if anyone else would blame me for not finding him—if they did, not a single person talked to me about it—but I blamed myself, relentlessly. The overwhelming feeling of failure and worthlessness that took residence in my body began to bury me. Without realizing it, I had thrown my heart into a dungeon where no one could hear its screams for help.

I talked about this fire continuously for weeks, searching for someone to admit to me that everyone else thought I'd fucked up, that I did something horrible and wrong, but no one did. I felt alone, like I carried a horrible secret.

Most first responders engage in what mental health professionals call "magical thinking." This means we believe if only we had done something different, we would have saved a life. We believe this even when we have nothing to do with the outcome. So many of us have built our self-worth from the job and being a rescuer. If we cannot rescue someone, our inner voices tell us it was our fault, even if there was absolutely nothing we could do.

Searching for a person in a fire is difficult. While the fire is burning and the building/room is full of smoke, you cannot see your hand in front of your face. Becoming disoriented happens fast. Firefighters have been found dead, unable to orient themselves to get out of a closet. We try to map a way out by keeping our shoulder against a wall. Meanwhile, kids and sometimes adults hide to be able to get out of the smoke and heat, making finding them even more difficult. Sometimes we don't find a person until after the fire when the smoke clears. Sometimes we even realize we've stepped or crawled over a body many times and never knew it.

But there was no fire by the time I was searching, and that's why my mistake was so inexcusable. The fire was out, the smoke was cleared, and the white linoleum kitchen floor contrasted with the darkly clothed person. I beat myself up for not finding that person. My inner voice constantly told me I'd fucked up and cost that man his life.

The reality, of course, was Truck 5 and Engine 5 had searched for this guy, too and couldn't find him. He was most likely dead before anyone had arrived on scene. Still, my magical thinking told me I should have found him. The box barely had room for this dead guy wrapped in magical thinking. I tried and tried but it would not fit in.

It was the beginning of the school year, so the UC Berkeley fraternities and freshmen dorms were in full swing, with plenty of drunken mayhem and vomiting. The freshman, away from answering to their parents' guidance and rules for the first time, do everything their parents wouldn't let them do at home. It felt like the movie Groundhog Day—and I became angrier with each passing day. My fuse shortened to a nub, and my temper blew quick. Everything at Station 3 that had previously annoyed me now infuriated me. I could not escape the heaviness of constant exhaustion or the aggravation of constant noise.

At forty-four years old, I had been in this line of work full time for twenty-five years. The distant ringing of an overflow alarm sounded inside my head. Day by day, the noise grew louder and grittier. Attempting to cram the dead guy into the box in my head had caused it to overfill. I desperately tried to gather the spilling contents and shove everything back inside and close the lid, but the contents continued to erupt out of the box.

For the first time in my life, I became completely over-whelmed and could not control my ribbon. I knew I had a problem, but I had no idea of its magnitude.

PART II

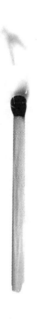

CHAPTER SEVENTEEN

It was February 2014, and seven months had gone by since the fire with the dead guy. The battle to fit all that crap back into the box became a losing battle. My chest constantly rattled with butterflies on drugs. My body shook with agitation, and the smallest irritation sent me into a rage. I couldn't see what went on around me. Newer firefighters who didn't know me well avoided me.

I sat with a firefighter and gave him his performance review.

When we were done, he said, "This is the first real review I have gotten while being here. So far they've all been pencil-whipped. I want to thank you for the good review. I thought you were going to rip me a new asshole."

I asked, "Why would I do that? You are a good at your job and you take pride in it."

"Well, you sure do yell at us a lot. You're always mad at us for something."

"Really?"

"Yeah."

"Well I promise to take a look at that."

In a panic, I called Wyatt, a coworker friend of mine, who seemed to have the pulse on everything going on at the department.

"Dude, my probie just told me I yell at everyone all the time. Is this real or is he just being sensitive?"

He said back, "It's true. And it's not just a coincidence that people are moving out of your station."

"But I totally take care of my crews."

"Yes, you do. No one disagrees with that. They just are tired of getting yelled at."

I hung up the phone and thought, *Well fuck me. That's not the captain I want to be. What is wrong with me? I need to fix this! Whatever "this" is.*

I realized Wyatt was right. My firefighters and medics were leaving to work at other stations when an opportunity arose. *What an absolute failure I am as a captain.* All I wanted was for everyone to be the best they could be. I never intended to hurt anyone. I knew good leaders didn't use shame. They inspired others to be better.

I realized later I had shamed everyone for the qualities I saw as weak—laziness, sloppy and inefficient work, and lack of physical and emotional strength. These were traits I feared I had. I had always held a contempt for myself deep down, and not finding the guy had brought that contempt to the surface. Now shame sprayed out of me and all over everyone who didn't rise high enough.

I had reached a tipping point. I had to figure out what the hell was going on and fix it.

The idea of leaving Engine 3 never crossed my mind. I had pride for this station where few people wanted to work because of the call volume. Engine 3 was destroying me from the inside. Yet I was not going to wimp out and move to another station. I knew all the nuances of this district—the houses with difficult access, the many blocked streets, the commercial building layouts, the good hydrants, the bad hydrants, etc. I couldn't leave the residents who lived here. If something happened in a tricky part of this district after I left, I would feel responsible. My stubbornness bound me to this station.

One evening, I stood in the kitchen cooking dinner for the crews when the station phone rang. "Hey Christy, this is Bobby. Those of us down at shift-bid headquarters are doing a mock bid, and we have you going to Station 6."

"Ha, ha, you are hilarious. Why would I leave Station 3?"

"Because you hate it there and have put up with all the bull-shit that goes along with three's district long enough. You need a change."

"But I know every inch of this district. The potential for huge incidents are all over this area. Besides, Nablooms Bakery is right next door, and I finally got them to stop having live bands play all night long."

"Well I implore you to seriously think about it. You need to leave and this is your opportunity. All of us at Station 2 think you should move to Station 6."

"I'll think about it but I am pretty sure I ain't going anywhere."

That same night, we ran seven calls after midnight. In the morning I climbed into my car and pulled out of the station driveway feeling like I'd been awake for two days straight because I had been.

Maybe Bobby Law is right, I thought. *I could use a change. Get off the treadmill.*

Engine 6 had its own challenges but no university dorms. No fraternities. No five-thousand-square-foot houses. Very few houses in that district were chopped into thirty apartments. No hills. No wildland area. Engine 6 covered the northwest corner of Berkeley. It was flat. The streets were wide. There were hydrants everywhere. The houses were single-story and small. A quarter of the district was industrial and warehouses, which meant people left the area to go home at night.

By the time I pulled into my driveway, I'd decided to make the move.

I started at Station 6 in March 2014. I came into the job knowing I needed to tone it down and be kind. I wanted to exemplify the leadership I'd always admired. I had a great crew who cared about their jobs and doing them well. I had an eager new driver and a seasoned firefighter who made me laugh all the time. They were compassionate toward the residents and treated everyone with respect. Rarely did I have to follow up with them. We ate dinner together and hung out during down time. I could count on these guys.

Within the first week after the move, I was feeling happy I'd made the change. At Station/Engine 6, the presleep, preplan only took a few minutes. I slept more and ran fewer calls. I hoped these changes meant my quick temper would ease, and my constant complaining would go away.

We ran plenty of calls, but they weren't the same needless calls over and over. There was no ambulance at Station 6, no bakery or alley next door . . . only a train horn blowing as it passed through the west end of Berkeley.

Soon, I started waking up before the sun. Like early. Like 4:30 a.m. early, wide-awake ready to start my day. At work, I found myself tiptoeing the halls of Station 6 while my crew continued to sleep.

At first, I thought, *This is pretty nice! Maybe I really don't need very much sleep!* But soon enough, I started not being able to fall asleep at work. If we didn't run calls during a forty-eight-hour shift, we had the same daily routine as one would have at home. We ate lunch around noon, dinner around 6:00 p.m., and went to bed in the late evening. We started our day around 7:00 a.m.

I'd usually try to crawl into bed around 10:00 p.m. Just like at home, I'd read for a bit then fall asleep. But now falling asleep took hours.

The anxiety began. The red lights in the ceiling lit up, and the speaker came to life. I'd hear "Engine 6," followed by a dispatcher sending us somewhere to face something. My heart pounded so hard I was sure everyone could see it through my shirt. It didn't matter how simple a call it might be, just the lights and tones sent a surge through my nervous system. I couldn't breathe, my chest hurt, and my legs felt like wet noodles. I could not control my ribbon. The panic pounded its way into every single part of me. I struggled to make sure no one would hear the waver in my voice or see my heart pounding.

I googled, "How to Control Your Body's Response to Stress." I found suggestions like "Close your eyes and breathe. Concentrate on something in the room." I couldn't close my eyes and sit still and concentrate on my breath. I had to hurriedly go save someone's life or their house. My desperation for answers continued to grow, but I couldn't tell anyone. If my coworkers knew I felt panic when the tones went off or if I showed any fear or weakness, I would become a fraud.

Then my sleep disappeared. At bedtime, exhaustion sent me right to sleep, but an hour later hypervigilance woke me. I'd rearrange my pillows and roll onto my stomach, then my side, then my other side. With each turn, I grew more annoyed and my tossing and turning became more aggressive. I'd look at the clock and as an hour or two would slowly pass by, I'd grow angrier.

After months of this, I accepted sleep would be rare.

At home, before I went to bed, I'd pile a stack of clothes on the corner of my dresser. I woke up around 4:00 a.m. every morning and quietly grabbed my stack of clothes without waking up Lisa.

Being wide awake so early felt like falling into another dimension. It was similar to driving into work on Christmas morning. No one would be on the road, as if a catastrophe had transpired overnight, and I was the only person left alive. I'd get up in the morning and be perplexed and alone, surrounded by the early-morning darkness and silence.

Soon enough, the videotape started playing. My brain created a montage of wretched calls I had been on that played in a loop that ran all . . . day . . . long. I could not stop it, just like a miserable song that took residence in someone's head.

My videotape was a horror show. The husband and wife who were ejected from their car. The screaming boy whose mom was dead in the front seat. The mother beaten to death by her husband with a fire poker in front of their four-year-old son. The professor run over by a truck and the devastated driver. The mother's scream when she was told her four-month-old was dead. The elderly woman whose burned skin came off on my turnouts as I carried her. The limp, gray guy I'd failed. They played over and over in my head.

My desperation grew. How was I going to fix this?

I continued to work. I continued to wake up every hour and not sleep. I continued to feel my heart pound through my chest every time the dispatch lights and tones went off. The videotape continued to play in my head and haunt me. Running a call was the only thing that shifted my brain out its shitty loop. But with fewer calls to run, the relief didn't come often.

Everything frustrated me. I wanted to punch holes in walls. I had a collection of smashed tennis rackets in my closet from the past few months. I ran hot with anger waiting to surface, ready to blow. I constantly wanted to fight. My ribbon exploded into my heart, drastically increasing my heart rate and latching onto my vocal cords so I could barely talk.

Most of my childhood and my adolescence I worked hard to overcome many obstacles and fix whatever the problem was in order to take care of myself and be successful. This time I couldn't. No matter what I did, I couldn't turn off the video or get any sleep. I couldn't stop the anxiety that put its hands around my throat. The symptoms became a part of everything.

Then the crying started. Oh dear Lord, the crying! I had never been a crier unless I got insanely angry. But now I started crying all the goddamn time.

I made an appointment with the same therapist I had seen several years ago to help me deal with some issues that were coming up around my mom. My plan was to identify what in the hell was going on, fix it, and be normal again.

Normal for me, of course, meant not being weak. It meant stopping the bullshit anxiety every time the tones went off. I was sure therapy would work. I'd spend a few months learning a few breathing exercises and techniques to relax, and then everything would be fine.

Lisa wanted to come with me for support. While I experienced shame for having a problem I couldn't handle on my own, I was thankful she supported me and still wanted to be with me. She never asked for help. Even when she had to go to the ER, I found out about it later.

We sat in the waiting room, and Lisa flipped through a magazine. I fidgeted in my chair. My therapist, Grace, was ten minutes late. Shrinks were never supposed to be late. *This is bullshit. I get my fifty minutes or an hour and then get cut off? What is the deal with this lady?* I stared at the floor, fuming.

The door finally opened and Grace stood in the doorway

while another lady walked out. Grace had a warm and comforting smile on her face as she waved me in.

I couldn't believe her audacity. Shouldn't she be apologizing instead of smiling? Clearly, she didn't give a shit she was late.

I walked into her bright office with wall-to-wall windows overlooking an upper layer of oak trees that lined the street outside. I sat down on her comfortable couch while she sat in a chair across from me. Her presence filled the entire room with kindness and refuge. Nothing distracted her. All her attention fell on me. All my gritty anger dissolved.

While clutching a pillow, I said, "Something is wrong with me."

"Okay, tell me what's going on," she said, with genuine compassion in her eyes.

"I can't sleep. I have a videotape of shitty calls I've run over the years that continuously plays in my head. I wake up from nightmares, screaming and drenched in cold sweat. I blow up over little things. Unless someone is what I think they should be, I treat them like shit. Whenever the tones go off at work for a call, my insides fold in half and it feels like my stomach has been turned inside out. And that's for any call. The tones can go off for a leaking hydrant and my body turns to mush."

Grace listened intently as I rambled on, angry because this bullshit should not be happening. Finally, I ran out of words.

"It sounds like you have PTSD," she said matter-of-factly.

A few silent moments passed, just the two of us looking at each other. I quickly decided I was going to pretend I didn't hear what she'd just said. I couldn't have PTSD. Soldiers who'd been in combat hell got PTSD. Weak people who couldn't handle this job got PTSD. Not me. No fucking way.

When my session ended, I walked out of Grace's office full of a mix of anger and disbelief. Lisa's eye met mine; tears welled in my eyes and I just kept walking.

Lisa got up and followed me out. Neither of us said a word until we got into my car. While staring straight ahead, I said, "She says I have PTSD."

Lisa reached over and put her hand on mine. We remained quiet all the way home.

I saw Grace every week after that. It cost me $140 every session out of pocket. I could go to EAP (Employee Assistance Program) through work for free, but we only got a few sessions. And while I knew it was supposed to be confidential, I couldn't risk it. No one at work could know. I would pay and do whatever I needed to do.

Grace, being a former first responder, understood. She had been a cop before becoming a therapist, and she'd spent ten years of the early part of her adult life as a cop in a gnarly city. I knew she was the real deal. This lady was smart and strong. She'd left law enforcement because she'd begun to see what that job could do to a person and had to get out before she became hardened and angry.

I felt safe with her. I somehow knew she wouldn't judge me. Ever. But I also felt like such a fake . . . like I was pretending to be this strong, fearless firefighter and if anyone knew the actual piece of shit I was inside, my cover would be blown. I would be the unlovable loser I always knew I was.

I was tired of being alert and "ready to go" at all times. When I walked into any building, whether I was at work or off duty, I'd size up the fuel load inside. I would look to see whether the building had fire sprinklers and where the exits were. I would plan how to get someone who was with me out. At home before I crawled to bed, I put everything away. I made sure the recliners were not reclined creating an obstacle to escaping in the middle of the night. I slid the screen door open so if we needed to bail out of the sliding glass door, there would be nothing to slow us down.

I had to keep moving. I could not sit still. Everything about my state of mind became unsurmountable. I worried I would be finished, have nothing, and be no one. In those moments, a new loop of catastrophizing overwhelmed me. *I am haunted. I am paralyzed. I am sick of myself. I am alone.*

After three sessions, Grace made a suggestion. "Since I am not an MD, I can't officially diagnose you. Why don't you go see a psychiatrist so you can get an official diagnosis? And maybe you can talk about medication."

I needed an "official" PTSD diagnosis in case I wanted to file a workers' compensation claim or take any time off work.

A few days later, Lisa and I sat in a psychiatrist's waiting room. I was nervous as fuck. My body continued to search for a comfortable position in my chair.

Finally, the doctor came out to get me and I walked into the meticulously decorated and spacious office. She asked me many questions about my symptoms. When I mentioned the looping calls that played in my head, she immediately wanted to know more.

I only got into the description of a few calls before she held up her hand.

"Wait, wait, wait. Stop," she said. "I don't want to hear anymore. If I do, I'll get PTSD. Yes, you have PTSD. Good God . . . what you have seen."

"That was only a couple of hours out of twenty-five years," I said truthfully.

"Let's talk about medication," she pivoted. "I think Zoloft would be good."

"Sure," I said, with no intention of ever taking it.

Afterward, as soon as Lisa and I got in the car, she pointed to my prescription and said, "Let's drop that off at the pharmacy on the way home."

Looking in the rearview mirror and backing out of the parking space, I said, "I'll do it later. I'm not going to start it till I get back from my trip."

The next day I would be getting on an airplane with a very good friend to Salt Lake City. I'd been asked to play on a team for a hockey tournament.

"Yeah," she said in her level tone, "you're going to drop it off now, though. That way it'll be ready when you come home."

Lisa knew if I had reluctance toward something, I'd procrastinate and spend forever sidestepping a way around it. And I knew Lisa would continue to push until I got this done.

"Fine," I said, and I steered the car to the pharmacy.

When I handed the pharmacist the prescription for Zoloft, I thought, *This is ridiculous. I need to explain myself. I can only imagine what this pharmacist thinks of me. She probably thinks I'm another one of those pathetic people who pull the stress card because they don't want to work.* I desperately wanted her to know my story, but I said nothing, praying no one would say "Zoloft" out loud for other people to hear.

Lisa made me go back the next day to pick up my bottle of weakness.

The morning after I returned from my trip, I took one dose of Zoloft. My stomach became queasy, and my head was dopey the rest of the day.

Enough of that. What was I thinking? I told Lisa I would never take meds.

CHAPTER EIGHTEEN

During the month of July, whenever my regular forty-eight-hour shift was over, I would get in my car, pull out of the station driveway, and start crying. I would cry all the fuck the way home. As I pulled into my driveway, a concerned Lisa would open the front door and see my wet face and red eyes.

"Don't worry," I'd say. "I'll be fine."

When I was off from work with my schedule of two days on and four off, I'd isolate myself and stew in anger and anxiety. I would run to prevent myself from blowing up. Running worked like a pressure relief valve. It never got rid of the anxiety or anger, it just quieted it. I would rally and then return to work. This cycle repeated itself every week.

I also continued to go to therapy once a week. Grace encouraged me to find some compassion for myself and recognize I was not a failure.

At work, I pretended like everything was normal. The only colleague I talked to was Jack. I had a tremendous amount of respect for Jack as a firefighter, paramedic, and person, and he'd experienced what I was going through.

A couple of years earlier, Jack had worked two significant fires a few days apart. In the first fire, he'd almost lost his life, and in the second fire, someone who he'd been trying to save didn't make it. I completely understood why he'd taken an entire year off.

My situation is totally different, I told myself. *Those calls were so much worse.*

Still, I sought him out as the sole person I confided in about what I was going through. During training, I pulled him aside, and we talked in hushed voices.

He looked me straight in the eyes one day and said, "You need to call Linda Brown (a workers' comp attorney). Fill out the paperwork and go home. Now." He pointed at my head. "You can't get your head straight while you're piling more on. You have to clean off your plate and deal with the mess in the middle."

I immediately protested, despite myself. "But Jack, I'm better than this. I should be able to handle it. You went through two horrific calls. I haven't done shit. This can't happen to me."

Jack pointed at my heart in my chest and said, "You are human. This can happen to you. Go fill out your paperwork and go home."

"There's no way I am going home now. They'd have to call someone in from home," I said, reflexively crossing my arms in front of me.

Jack shook his head. "Well suit yourself, but I'm telling you, you need to call Linda Brown and take some time off."

Grace also urged me to take some time off. Still, I resisted.

Then my reaction to the tones at work escalated even more. I began to dread them going off and sending me to a family involved in a gruesome car accident on the freeway. Instead of compassion, pressurized steam and outrage would fill me. I envisioned what the scene would look like. With gritted teeth and muscles wound tight, I would move about the car wreck pulling them out of their mangled car, securing those that lived to backboards and covering those that didn't with a yellow blanket. I would take good care of them, but I'd cuss under my breath at them for putting me here again. Any call I attended to was adding to the already-full box in my head. Knowing that at any second, I might be sent on another horrible call, made me feel like I was being buried alive and suffocating in anxiety.

I finally agreed to take a break.

I had some time off coming up. I was going to play in a hockey tournament and see my dad in Oregon. If I could get a couple more days off in between those trips, I'd get four weeks off. I made some desperate phone calls. Drew and another guy were kind enough to trade shifts with me at the last minute. This meant I owed them, but it also meant I'd get a much-needed reprieve from the dread that sat on me like a heavy blanket.

With a level of doom hanging over me, I knew what was coming, and I made the call to Linda Brown, the workers' compensation attorney.

My colleagues referred to Linda Brown as a bulldog, though I know she didn't like the reference. She was tall, thin, and blond, and, well, a bulldog, but with a gigantic heart. Linda Brown represented mostly first responders, including some of my coworkers from Berkeley Fire. I had met her through presentations she'd given to my department on workers' comp. She gave us general advice and ways we could get the best care within the workers' comp system.

If someone didn't follow her advice and then asked for help, I don't know how else to say this but she would rip that person a new one. Luckily, I had followed all her instructions before any of this happened. I had no doubt when Linda Brown walked into a courtroom. The opposing lawyer dropped his pen in defeat, knowing he'd soon be conceding to her demands.

The day I finally called her for help, her receptionist told me she was out of town.

"No hurry," I said. "Really no hurry at all."

A wave of relief hit as I got to kick the can farther down the road. Linda was unavailable, and I was heading to Las Vegas to play in an ice hockey tournament. Some of my favorite people and my favorite activity awaited me in Vegas—six friends and four ice hockey games in three days, plus, alcohol, lots of food, and an enormous amount of laughter. These people all loved me, and it was just the medicine I needed.

After meeting up with my friends in Vegas, the first item on the agenda was acquiring beer, whiskey, snacks, Gatorade, and water at the grocery store. My friends and I walked in and I headed off in my own direction.

While walking down the chips and cookies aisle, my phone rang and I answered.

"Is this Christine Warren?"

"Yes."

"This is Linda Brown."

Holy shit! Linda Brown was calling me. Hope and relief came in and lifted some weight off my shoulders. And she made it much easier by calling me and offering her support instead of me having to call again and asking for it.

"I got your message," she said, "and I wanted to tell you that anyone who can admit to me they have PTSD is going to get my help. I know this is an awful thing you're going through, but you will not be alone. I'll be with you every step of the way."

Just then, a young, perfectly manicured man in his perfect blue uniform and shiny Las Vegas Firefighter badge came around the corner, pushing a grocery cart. I stared, thinking, *Dude, you have no idea what you are getting yourself into.* I felt sorry for the guy. I wanted to tell him what could happen, but I just shook my head and thought, *Poor fucker.*

"Linda I cannot thank you enou—"

"We'll take care of this, okay? Call the office and make an appointment. Now I'm getting off the phone."

I heard the *click* as she hung up, but I was a little less alone than before. I now had the largest, most caring, smartest, fearless combatant fighting for me.

Removing the heavy weight of work from my shoulders did give me some relief, as I'd hoped, and when I came back to Station 6 four weeks later on September 11, 2014, I actually looked forward to going back to work.

We were scheduled for training in the morning. Since our drill tower and classroom were onsite, we walked over. I called dispatch on the radio to put us out of service for training. The three of us headed next door along with half the department. All fourteen of us wore the same blue wool outfits and meandered around the classroom, chatting until we were told to get started.

Just before 8:46 a.m., the time the planes hit the first tower, we formed a circle around the flag in the memorial garden at Station 6. We bowed our heads in silence to honor and reflect on the events and those we lost on that day. The garden area remained still and silent except for the constant sound of cars driving up and down Cedar Street outside the fence.

Our meditation was interrupted by a crash followed by, "*Aaaarrgghhhh!*"

We lifted our heads up and looked at each other. Without saying a word, all fourteen of us filed out of the garden. In the middle of the street, a bicyclist lay on the ground in front of a stopped car.

Someone better take charge, I thought to myself, and just as quickly, I realized this was my district, so I was the person to take charge. We all sprang to action. I got on the radio to tell dispatch to send an ambulance and BPD. I told my driver, who'd already began moving in that direction, to pull the rig out and block traffic in front of us. The medics in the group attended to the bicyclist, whose arm was clearly broken. The driver and a young kid remained in their car.

I helped them get out of their car and onto to the sidewalk. Tears rolled down both of their faces.

"Is he going to be okay?" the driver asked.

"He's going to be fine," I assured her. "He just has a broken arm."

A few witnesses had stopped to tell their account of watching him run the stop sign.

"There is nothing you could have done," I told her. "He earned his own broken arm. This is on him. Not you in anyway."

I turned to the kid and bent down, "You okay? I know this is scary, but everything is gonna be fine. You guys did nothing wrong. He ran right out in front of you with no warning. He'll get a cast and his friends will get to sign it and everything will be all right, okay?"

The kid nodded, "Okay," through his tears.

Normally, there would be five people on scene, and each person would have a pre-determined task. In this case, there were sixteen of us. We ran the call smoothly and precisely. Everyone took a task and completed it. The medics loaded the bicyclist into the ambulance and headed to the hospital. My driver backed the engine into the station. We picked up our trash and headed back to the classroom.

I took four steps and started crying.

Before having PTSD symptoms, I had never cried at work, unless I was extremely angry. Everything on this call had gone well. I was proud of the job we'd all done, and this was no big deal. *What in the fuck is wrong with me?*

I yelled to my firefighter, "I gotta run in the station real quick. I'll be over in a second."

I headed to the bathroom, shut the door, splashed some water on my face, and tried to regain my composure. I then walked back to the classroom and quietly sat down in the back row, thinking, *This is unacceptable.*

CHAPTER NINETEEN

On Monday, October 6, 2014, the air in Berkeley buzzed with the start of the work week. My long shift of thirty-four hours on, fourteen off, and forty-eight on had finally ended. I told myself, *If I just keep my shit together and don't cry on the way home, I'm going to be fine.*

I took apart my bed, hung my uniform up, and put my steel-toed boots away in my locker. Pictures of those I loved and drawings from my nieces lined my locker door. The captain who was on duty after me showed up to relieve me. I put my turnouts, helmet, and axe back in the rack labeled "WARREN." The oncoming captain and I discussed the happenings of the prior two days, and I waved a goodbye. "Have a good four-day," I said to my crew and a "Have a safe shift," to the oncoming crew. I started up my car and pulled out of the driveway. I took a deep breath and thought to myself, *I can do this.*

As I drove home, I concentrated on the words "do not cry." As I passed through the Caldecott Tunnel, where my emotions tended to overwhelm me, I focused even more. *Do not cry.* And I didn't. I made it all the way home without crying. I didn't cry as I drove through the city of Berkeley, through the Caldecott Tunnel, along Highway 24, and the rest of the way home. I pulled into my driveway doing a mental fist pump. *Success! I did it!*

I was going to be okay. As long as I focused, I could do this. I got my work bag out of my car and walked into the house like I had just won a championship game. The dirty clothes of the last several days went into the laundry hamper.

I sent my wife a text. "I did it. I made it all the way home without crying. I'm good!"

I had a tennis date with a friend, so I changed my clothes, grabbed my tennis stuff, and cruised out the door.

Still infused with the high of making it home without falling apart, I drove down the street looking for something to listen to on the radio. I wasn't really focusing on anything.

And that's when it hit. Hard. Without warning, the scenes and shitty memories flooded back. I couldn't turn it off. They hit harder and brighter, with the volume louder than ever before. It was like being trapped in a movie theater with a wretched movie playing where I couldn't close my eyes or turn my head away. Tears streamed down my face, which became sobbing. I punched the car door. *What in the fuck?*

A pole came into view. I imagined pushing the accelerator to the floor, hearing the engine rev up, and seeing the pole come closer and closer until a huge collision sent glass flying and metal twisting. I saw my eyes close, and my body sit limp in the driver's seat.

No, a pole was no good. Poles were designed to fall over when hit. That wouldn't do the job. What I needed was a tree. A tree would do the job. I wouldn't have to go back to work and no one would ever find out what a complete failure I was. Even if I ended up in the hospital for a couple of months, I could just lie there in a medically induced coma and not have this crap in my head. I'd get a break and wouldn't have to feel any of this bullshit. I wouldn't have to confess to anyone just how deep a weakness resided within me.

I barely made it to the tennis courts without steering myself into a tree. The thought of how I'd just be adding to more first responders' pile of shitty calls if I did that was a big part of what got me there safely.

Before getting out of the car, I texted Lisa, "You cannot let me go back to work. No matter how much I beg and plead and how stubborn I am and say I am fine after the four-day, you must not let me go back."

She texted back, "I had already made that decision."

That afternoon, I made the call to the battalion chief on duty.

"Hey, Frank," I said, as casually as I could manage. "How do I turn in workers' comp paperwork for a cumulative injury where I can't go to work right now?"

Frank answered, "Do you need to be seen by a doctor?"

"I don't know," I said vaguely. "I guess so."

"What's it for?" he asked.

I hesitated. "PTSD."

Frank replied, "Oh, okay. Let me call the chief and see exactly how he wants this done. Can I call you right back?"

When he called back a minute later, he asked if I'd be willing to turn my paperwork into the fire chief and talk to him. I agreed. I knew the fire chief well. He ran my academy, and I'd worked for him when he was a captain and I was a paramedic.

Before we hung up, Frank said, "If you need anything or someone to talk to, just let me know."

The next morning, October 7, I drove to Berkeley and had to look for a place to park in front of the fire administration building. I walked up the stairs in my civilian clothes into the fire chief's office. He closed the door, and I handed him my paperwork in defeat.

We sat down at his round table—and I started fucking crying.

"This is the hardest thing I have ever done in my entire life," I said. "To admit that I cannot do my job, too weak to show up at work, is absolutely killing me inside. I'm sorry for letting the department down."

For a long moment, he stared at me with a baffled expression. "Do you know what happened? Was it the responsibility of being a captain?"

"I honestly don't know," I said. "I plan on fixing this and getting better. I plan on coming back and being a battalion chief someday."

He continued to sit with his hands clasped together on top of the table, his eyes wide open, confused. "Well, okay," he said, "just make sure you take care of yourself."

I managed to turn off the tears and look right into his eyes. "I *will* be back," I said firmly, even as defeat ran through my body, crushing my heart.

Failure chased me out of the building as I hurriedly walked down the hallway, wishing I could run. Just before opening the door to the outside, I stopped to pull myself together again. I dreaded I'd see an engine pull up and have to face someone I know or anyone in uniform who was strong enough to continue to do the job. The thought of everyone knowing what a failure I was ate me up inside. *I can't leave my job and the department like this.*

I resolved to take some time off, get my shit together, and come back as if nothing had happened.

Four days later, on October 10, Lisa and I sat in two chairs in front of Linda Brown's reception desk. I'd tried to insist I drive the fifty-minute drive to her office, but Lisa won that argument. I didn't get why she wanted to drive, but as soon as we reached the heart of Vallejo and I could see Highway 37, I understood.

All the fatal wrecks came flooding back, and I proceeded to fold in half and started crying.

"Thank you for driving," I mumbled.

"You're welcome." Lisa was a calm and steady presence, her support unwavering for me, even as I made life so difficult for her.

I had become irrational. The level of how upset I got with her in no way matched whatever the incident was that would set me off. Normally, arguing was a rarity—fighting never. Now, I'd start arguments that left us both in tears and me begging her not to leave me, even though she never floated the idea that she might.

Once we got beyond Highway 37, I was able to breathe again.

At Linda Brown's office, the receptionist offered us tea, coffee, or water.

We both politely declined and sat down to wait.

Lisa flipped through a magazine, and I stared. I was scared. I had no idea what I feared, but the dread flooded through my body. My stomach twisted, making me nauseous. I quickly scanned the room for a trash can.

After waiting for about ten minutes, a tall blond woman, bent forward at her shoulders, marched across the room toward us. She immediately pointed at us and said to the receptionist, "Did you offer these guys anything?" You would have thought she was from New York, given her demeanor and attitude. She always told you exactly what she felt and thought, and she was sarcastic.

I loved her, although she infuriated me occasionally.

"She did, I promise," I said hastily. "We are good."

"Well, then, let's go into my office!"

We followed her into her small office and sat in two chairs very close to her desk. Her office was filled with firefighting and police trinkets, which clients had given her over the years. My eyes settled on pictures of someone riding a horse. Small trophies with horses lined a shelf on the wall behind her. Behind her sat stacks and stacks of case files.

Linda talked, but I could not listen. My eyes welled up, and I lowered my forehead so it rested on the edge of her desk.

"What are you crying about?" she asked in disbelief, interrupting whatever she'd been attempting to convey to me. "We haven't even started talking about anything. Geez, you got it bad."

Lisa had brought a notebook and paid close attention on my behalf, writing things down. I continued not to hear most of what Linda said. At some point, I realized they'd moved onto a different topic.

"Are you two married?" Linda asked. "Like legally married?"

"Yes, we are."

"Good, because if you weren't, they could force Lisa to testify against you. You two wouldn't be protected, and Lisa wouldn't have the attorney-client privilege."

Lisa and Linda went over the to-do list. Lisa would later make sure I did everything Linda said, since for me much of this conversation just didn't sink in.

As we wrapped things up, Linda's face softened with kindness, and said, "You feel like you've failed every single female firefighter, huh?"

"Yes, that's exactly how I feel."

"I figured," she said. "Do you have any plans to kill yourself? Because I'm not going to waste my time if you are just going to go off yourself. Do you hear me?"

"I'm not gonna to do anything," I said with an undertone of trying to make her happy.

"Do you have a gun?"

"Yes."

"What kind?"

"A Glock 9mm."

Exasperated, she threw her arms up in the air and said, "Oh, Jesus. Get that thing out of the house—do you understand me? You have too much to live for. Don't you dare. All right, now I'm done with you two." She shooed us out of her office.

In order to take time off work, I had to file a workers' compensation claim. The City of Berkeley used the workers' compensation company, ACS, to provide their workers' compensation insurance. ACS had notoriously been hard to deal with. They denied legitimate claims regularly. I knew this was going to be a small war.

Linda had rules she expected me to follow. I must always tell the truth and be nice to my claims adjuster, she had said, and we would win this case.

Following Linda's first rule would be simple, as I'm a consummate truth-teller. And as long as my adjuster didn't suggest I was faking all of this, she and I were going to be fine.

The first item on Linda's to-do list was going to see my workers' comp doctor.

"So, what seems to be the problem?" Dr. Smith asked, flipping through my chart.

I told him about the PTSD, nightmares, anxiety, and the videotape of horrible calls in my head.

"Were you harassed by someone?"

"No," I said, wondering about the relevance of his question.

"Was there a bad call that started all this?" he asked.

I told him about the night of the fatal fire, but I knew that was just the event that had blown the lid off, not the cause.

He furrowed his brow. "Isn't that something you do—like, isn't it part of your job?"

Dumbfounded, I said nothing.

"Well," he said, "if you can't do your job, then I guess you'll have to do light duty."

Panic welled inside of me to where my chest hurt. "I can't do light duty," I said. "I'll still be around all of it. I'll still have to wear my uniform and listen to the radios, hear all the sirens, and everything else associated with being a firefighter. I'll have to listen to my coworkers talking about calls. There's just no way."

"Well, I don't understand the problem, but whatever." He shrugged. "I'll put you off work and refer you to this lady . . . what's her name . . . Dr. Fong."

I couldn't believe him. I was in utter shock. He had always been so good to me during our annual department physicals. How could he suddenly be so disparaging, so dismissive? I felt like I had done something wrong, but I was pissed, too. Once I got the paperwork I needed from him, I stormed out without saying a word to anyone who worked there.

CHAPTER TWENTY

There were different treatment modalities for treating the symptoms of PTSD. Grace suggested I see an EMDR (eye movement desensitization and reprocessing) therapist in addition to seeing her. Now that I was off work, getting better was my full-time job.

I sat in another waiting room to confess to one more person that I was a weakling who couldn't do her job.

Caroline was a gracious woman with a kind smile. After a few sessions of getting to know me, we started the EMDR therapy. I held a buzzer in each hand while she asked me to talk about a particular incident that swirled in my head. She guided me through reframing each situation with the buzzers going, which was supposed to help me "reprocess" the memory and diminish the visceral response to it.

Caroline suggested a practice EMDR session on an upsetting event in my life outside of work. It worked perfectly. Before, I had felt extremely angry with someone, and after the session, the anger response disappeared. But when we tried EMDR sessions with the work incidents, the intensity of my responses never diminished.

When I complained to her that I was failing at EMDR, she gently corrected me.

"Christy, you cannot fail at EMDR. That's not how it

works." She explained sometimes while doing EMDR, the memory could feel very real, as if I was back in the specific spot. I did not experience any realness of a call. I wondered if EMDR would not be able to pull out the calls that were bolted to a certain part of my brain.

Sometimes during my therapy sessions when I talked, I didn't realize how much I was letting out the smelly messiness of my insides. Something inside would wake up and set off alarms, screaming, *Just shut the fuck up, Christy. Get your shit together.* Shame rose inside of me, urging me to stop sharing, stop the exposure. *No one is going to love me if they see what's really inside of me.*

Every time I came home from therapy, Lisa asked how it went. If I didn't want to talk about it, she didn't pressure me, but I could see my issues were wearing on her.

Worst of all was my hopelessness, which came with blinders. I could see nothing else. No matter the solution presented to me, I saw every issue as hopeless.

I didn't realize how much my despair was impeding any progress toward getting better. I couldn't see through the chaos in my head and the panic in my heart. It was like a record repeatedly skipping. I wanted to stop it, but I wouldn't let anyone near the needle to move it.

About two weeks after seeing Linda Brown, Lisa asked me if I'd filled out my disability insurance paperwork yet. When my sick and vacation leave ran out, I'd have no income. I would have to spend my savings, and when that ran out, dip into my retirement savings. Lisa knew that would add more stress to my already full plate and urged me to fill out the paperwork and turn it in.

"Not yet," I said, knowing I had no intention of filing a claim with my private disability insurance.

I recoiled from the word "disability." There was no way in hell I'd let someone call me disabled. I would rather be completely alone, broke, and eat nothing but peanut butter and jelly sandwiches than have to identify myself as disabled.

Besides, I could live off my retirement savings for a while. Meanwhile, letters from workers' comp, which were completely separate from the disability insurance, began to show up in my mailbox. Around the middle of October, two letters from workers' compensation landed in my mailbox. They might as well been written in a foreign language for how confusing they were.

October 16, 2014

You may lose your rights if you do not take certain actions within ten days. Read this letter and any enclosed fact sheets very carefully.

Dear Ms. Warren:

Acme Claim Solutions is handling your workers' compensation claim on behalf of the City of Berkeley. This notice is to advise you of the status of disability benefits for your workers' compensation injury on the date shown above.

Workers' compensation benefits are being delayed because we need to obtain additional information surrounding your claimed injury. Please provide medical evidence to support your claim as well as completion of the attached Injury Questionnaire and Medical Authorization forms within the next 30 days. If we do not receive these documents within this time frame, your claim will be denied.

We will notify you of our decision on or before 01/04/2015. Because this delay of benefits is related to a medical issue, enclosed with this notice is an informative fact sheet for your review.

In summary, they were telling me there would be a delay, and they were going to take as long as they needed to decide. If I hadn't had the means to pay out of my pocket to get help, I would have been navigating all this on my own, without any professional help. Fourteen days earlier, I'd almost killed myself by driving into a pole—and now they were going to take their time.

By the time first responders ask for help, they're already at the end of their rope. I needed help right now—not four months from now. Their disregard for this was infuriating.

The second letter from ACS stated I needed to get a psychological evaluation within thirty days. The letter listed the names of three doctors who could fit me in within that time frame. I called all three of them only to discover none of them could see me within thirty days. One even said he didn't have an appointment until February 10, 2015—four months away.

Panic began to spin inside me. What would it mean if I couldn't get an evaluation until after their imposed deadline?

I scrambled to figure out what my options were while I desperately tried to just get through each day. I was drowning in shame, lack of sleep, and anxiety, not able to work, while workers' comp stood on the shore, holding a life preserver and telling me they might throw it to me, or they might not. While being pulled underwater, I had to follow complicated instructions and articulately explain why I needed that life preserver.

The system felt set up to fail. Even if I didn't drown before the absolutely latest deadline came and they were instructed to throw me a lifeline, I knew they'd choose the cheapest, lowest quality life preserver they could find.

CHAPTER TWENTY-ONE

The last week of October, I had my first appointment with Dr. Fong. I arrived at her building and couldn't even decide where to park. I pulled in and out of at least four spots, searching for the best one. The first building I walked into, I couldn't find her office. I went into the other building and walked up and down the hallway until I found it. The ribbon surged through me, but instead of adrenaline and clarity, it consisted of frustration and anger.

I finally found her office and opened the door. A counter stood next to the door, and a woman behind it shuffled papers. I waited to be acknowledged.

Finally, after several minutes, she said, "Dr. Fong will be with you in a moment."

I continued to stand there.

A door across from me opened, and a woman emerged. She walked past me without acknowledging me. I stood there at the counter since there was no waiting area. I felt completely invisible, the same way I felt growing up. The same way I had felt my entire life.

My anger surged with each passing minute. After Dr. Fong walked past me a few times, I blew my top and yelled, "Obviously you don't have time for me and have other more important things to deal with, so screw this. I'm just going to leave."

I headed toward the door, but Dr. Fong put her hand on my arm and said, "No, I will be right with you. Go have a seat in my office."

I overflowed with anger and had to restrain myself from punching a hole in the wall. Walking through Dr. Fong's door was hard enough, but then to be disregarded like this was complete bullshit. I stomped into her office, sat in a chair in front of her desk, crossed my arms across my chest, and waited. I didn't realize I was holding my breath until I exhaled and there was barely any air to release.

Finally, Dr. Fong came in, closed the door, and sat behind her desk. She apologized for the waiting, shuffled some papers around her desk, and pecked away at her computer—apparently creating a file on me but saying nothing. This woman's communication and people skills were something to behold.

We exchanged some introductory conversation and then the questions began. She never looked away from her computer screen. "Tell me, how long have you been a firefighter and/or paramedic?" she said.

Leaning forward, looking right at her I answered, "Twenty-five years."

"What symptoms are you having?"

I leaned back in my chair. "I can't sleep. I'm racked with anxiety. I have a videotape of crappy incidents I've experienced on the job that play in my head continuously that I cannot turn off. I have a short fuse and blow pretty quick."

"Are you drinking?"

"Yes. A few drinks in the evening." I answered like it was no big deal.

She never asked how many drinks were "a few." But the truth was, these days I would drink only two drinks in front of Lisa, but as soon as she headed to the shower, I'd chug right out of a bottle of scotch or whiskey.

What is she doing? Filling out some questionnaire found in the back of a magazine? "Do you have PTSD? Take this quiz and find out."

"Who's taking care of household duties? Paying the bills and doing laundry and things like that?" she asked, still never glancing up from her computer.

"I dunno. I guess my wife is doing most of that at the moment," I said. I grew impatient with those rapid-fire questions.

"Are you suicidal?" She finally made eye contact with me.

"If you're asking if I wouldn't mind not being on this earth anymore, then yes, but I also don't have any plans to off myself at the moment."

Her gaze returned to her computer screen. The questions continued.

Finally, Dr. Fong stopped typing and looked directly at me. "Everything you have described is very typical for PTSD. You will continue to have these symptoms for a while. I'm going to take you off work for two months."

I had just been on shift-by-shift sick leave up to this point. To have two solid months off was definitely a step in the right direction. My annoyance at Dr. Fong softened slightly.

"I have no doubt you will be off for much longer," she said matter-of-factly, "but workers' comp will have a fit if I put you off for more than that at a time."

She filled out paperwork that formally stated I was unfit for duty for the next two months. Knowing I had a two-month reprieve loosened the grip around my throat and chest.

For now, I could breathe.

The entire month of October, I was too exhausted to sleep. Watching TV registered the same as watching a blank wall. My body flopped into bed feeling like lead weights, and yet I could not fall asleep. I'd become a container with nothing inside. Nothing could get through the thick coating of, "All I want is my job back."

Feelings of inadequacy overwhelmed me. When someone's house was burning down or someone was dying in front of me, only the task in front of me existed. Nothing else mattered. I didn't have the space to think about whether anyone loved me or how worthless I was. In that space, I'd always felt the most comfortable, my most alive. I'd gladly run into a burning building or help a severely injured person instead of sitting with myself.

My job was a perfect armor. It protected me and ensured I'd never be seen as weak. I wore a uniform with a badge of authority and protective garments such as steel-toed and shanked boots for my feet, turnouts for my body, gloves for my hands, and a helmet for my head. I even wore a bottle on my back and a mask on my face. In my fire gear, I breathed my own air.

Now my armor had been stripped from me, and I couldn't escape the parts of myself I'd avoided for so long.

By the middle of November, I still wasn't sleeping much. When I did fall asleep, I'd wake up an hour later. I'd wrestle with sleep all night until about 5:00 a.m., and I'd finally get up and tiptoe around the house so I didn't wake Lisa.

During what precious little time I slept, the nightmares got worse. One night I fell asleep and dreamed I was at work and my coworkers were there with me. They started running fast into a burning building. Somehow, I knew it was going to blow, so I screamed at them to stay back. They kept running. I ran after them, screaming for them to get back. But I was helpless, the building exploded, and I saw my fellow firefighters blown to bits.

I woke up screaming and fighting so hard. I flipped myself out of my bed and onto the floor.

Lisa woke up, startled, and asked, "Are you okay?"

I was on the floor, covered in sweat. "I'm fine."

Swearing under my breath, I got up off the floor and changed into dry pajamas. I most definitely was not fine.

CHAPTER TWENTY-TWO

Throughout November, I only focused on how my life used to be and how it had become so hopeless. I only saw what I didn't have.

One afternoon, I rode my indoor bike while I watched TV. I found and watched a show about the PJs, military rescue jumpers in Afghanistan. At first, I watched these guys with admiration, thinking, *I'd love to do that.* The admiration quickly deteriorated into shitty thoughts about myself, of how miserably weak I was. *Look at the crap these guys are dealing with, and they continue on! None of them are crying!* I continued to watch and berate myself. Finally, I climbed off the bike and headed to the liquor cabinet.

Unable to find an internal off switch in my head, I was increasingly turning to alcohol for comfort. No matter what I did, I couldn't move forward toward recovery. Instead, I was caught in a whirlpool of shame and darkness.

Grace tried to find something that would give me relief. She suggested taking medication for the depression, anxiety, and other PTSD symptoms. I refused. Taking medication would confirm my weakness, proving something was inherently wrong with me. She suggested bringing in a person who did a different type of therapy. I agreed to continue with EMDR, but I couldn't bring myself to tell yet another person how ridiculously weak I was. She even brought up finding a retreat/stay place to go. I said I didn't need to go to rehab.

I just wanted to be fixed so I could go back to work. At work, I did not have to face my worthlessness. At work, I was visible. Ironically, I was so used to being invisible that being out in public in uniform also made me uncomfortable. It was a constant push-pull—I so desperately wanted to be seen but when I finally was, fear and awkwardness took over. I was afraid someone would see the real, unworthy, unlovable me.

My work friends continued to text and call me. Every text and call was a gift, but I didn't call them back. I didn't know what to say. How could I admit to everyone I was a scam? How did I tell the very people whose respect I'd yearned for that I was a fraud? I had become the very thing I'd railed against for so many years. The captain had jumped ship. I couldn't think of anything more disgraceful.

If one of my crew were trapped in a fire, I would stay with them even if it meant my death. I would never leave them. But here I was, running away. I had absolutely nothing to give.

The nightmares continued. One night, I dreamed I was at work and somehow ended up at a pool party, still wearing my uniform. There were kids in the pool who were not good swimmers. They doggy paddled and clung to the sides. I mentioned something about the danger to the owner of the house and he snapped.

"You just mind your own business. Those kids are just fine."

I disagreed, and he blew up into a rage and told everyone to get out of the water. Kids begrudgingly climbed out and stood on the cement, water dripping off of them, pleading to go back in.

The angry host yelled, "No one is going back into that pool except for her!"

He tossed an infant into the pool. She hit the water and rapidly sank. I jumped in after her, but I couldn't break through the surface of the water. I had to save her. I was the rescuer, but I couldn't—no matter what I did. I watched the infant sink farther and farther down. I screamed in anger and frustration.

I woke up to Lisa frantically patting me, trying to hold my flailing arms and saying, "It's okay, it's okay." My sheets and pjs were soaked with cold sweat.

The next morning, Lisa casually mentioned to me, "One of us needs to sleep on the couch. I'm not getting any sleep with your nightmares. We can't both be exhausted."

I took a few seconds, then replied, "Fine. I get it. I'll sleep on the couch."

Lisa was right. For us to survive this, one of us had to have our wits about them. For Lisa to have the strength to take care of us and my shitshow, she had to get sleep.

I understood, but I also felt abandoned.

In November, I had a second meeting with Linda Brown, and she brought up the West Coast Post-Trauma Retreat, a six-day residential program that provides education, support, and healing designed to help active, former, and retired first responders recognize the signs and symptoms of posttraumatic stress injury in themselves and others.

Dr. Fong had mentioned this place as well. I agreed to look into it.

I sat down at my computer later that day to read up on the retreat. As I read the testimonials on their website, tears streamed down my face. *Holy shit, these people are describing exactly how I feel.*

After reading how this place had helped first responders

going through the same hell as me, I thought, *What the hell, I have nothing to lose. I need to try.*

I felt like I was the only firefighter in the world going through something like this. Reading other first responders' stories, it occurred to me for the first time that perhaps I wasn't alone in this.

At this point, I finally found some piece of strength and worked up the guts to call WCPR. I dialed the number, hesitating the entire time. As instructed per the recording, I left a message after the beep.

"Uh, hi . . . my name is . . . Christy Warren," I stammered. I explained who I was and that I wanted to come to the retreat. I hung up wondering if the place was real and if anyone would call back. There was a retreat scheduled for early December, which I hoped to get into.

The next morning, after another bout of nightmares and another morning full of pounding anxiety, I went on a run. The anxiety became desperate. I called Grace on her personal cell phone for help, something reserved for emergencies only. While waiting for her to call me back, I drove twenty minutes to the Lafayette Reservoir trail. Set back in the hills, trees and nature lined both sides of the trail, which wrapped around a lake. A light rain fell, my favorite running conditions. I set off running, carrying my phone with me.

One mile in, my phone rang. I stopped in my tracks. It wasn't Grace; it was Miles Pond, calling back from WCPR.

"Do you have time to talk?" he asked.

"Yes," I said. "I'm breathing fast cuz I'm on a run. I do want to talk to you, though."

Miles got right to the point. He asked, "Why do you think you need to come to WCPR?"

"Because I have PTSD and I'm a fucking mess," I said, as I paced back and forth in the rain. A middle-aged guy in amazing shape made eye contact with me as he ran by.

"Are you drinking?"

Looking at the ground, I replied, "Uh, yes. Not right this moment, but yeah, I have."

"How much?"

"Too much. I'd have a few drinks—hard liquor. And then when my wife went to take a shower, I'd drink out of the bottle. I realized I was drinking too much when I needed to buy some cheap whiskey cuz chugging straight out of an eighty dollar bottle of scotch was a waste. So I have stopped cold for a couple of weeks."

Two women passed me, deep in conversation. I hoped they hadn't heard me.

"Now, no bullshitting here," Miles said. "Have you thought about suicide?"

"A few times. I just want this shit out of my head."

"Tell me the worst three calls," he said.

"I don't think I can pick the top three. I have at least one hundred I could tell you about."

"Well, if there were three calls you could erase from your memory, what would they be?"

"We had a fire, and I fucked up and this guy ended up dying."

I then told him about the elderly woman I found and carried out of a fire and how her burned skin rubbed off on my turnouts. At the same time, a mom walked by with her twins in the stroller. She gave me a pained look, which implied, *Do you really need to talk about that here?*

I continued to pace back and forth on the trail.

More people passed by in opposing directions. One woman gave me a look of disgust.

Finally, Miles said he'd heard what he needed to hear and offered me a place at the retreat being held in March.

"March?" Having to wait four months kicked me in the gut. "Holy shit." The glimmer of hope that had begun to rise, disappeared. I needed to be at that retreat several months ago. I thought for sure he'd give me a spot in the December retreat just a couple of weeks out.

"Yeah, I know, I'm sorry, but that's the soonest I can get you in."

"Okay," I said, feeling more dejected than when I'd started my run.

"Sorry. Just keep running and seeing your therapist. If you need anything, please call me."

"Thank you, Miles"

Well, fuck me. March. I stood on the side of the trail in the rain with my hands on my hips. *I am not sure if I can make it that long. But at least Miles gets it.* A small but bright glimmer of hope shot through me.

Maybe I'm not the only one.

I hadn't talked to my family much about my situation. I'd only told them I was off from work because I had PTSD. When I emailed my dad, he replied, "I'm sorry you have to deal with this." The questions that followed were all about work and income, things already weighing on me.

But the evening of my conversation with Miles Pond, my dad called.

"*60 Minutes* just did a story on veterans with PTSD," he said. "Some veterans talked about suicide. Um . . . ah . . . do you ever get feelings like that or think like that?"

My dad had never asked me a question about my feelings. Our interactions had always lived on the surface. If I ever tried to talk about deeper feelings and thoughts, he would quickly bring it back to how he thought or his experience with something, never hearing a word I said.

But now he was asking if I'd been suicidal. I was grateful because I felt he cared. The concern in his heart moved right through to me in his voice.

"Ya. I've had those feelings. But really, please don't worry. I'll be fine. I won't ever do it. I just get the thoughts."

CHAPTER TWENTY-THREE

In early December, Lisa and I had been watching the news regarding the recent Berkeley protests in response to the police shootings in Ferguson.

I said to her, "Charles from Engine 6 texted today to see how I was doing. He told me about a 911 call they couldn't get to in time due to the blocked streets. The guy died in front of them. Such fucking bullshit."

Even though I wasn't on the call, my emotions were so close to the surface, I started crying. I realized I never wanted to feel what those guys felt ever again, but at the same time, I wanted to go back to work. Working again invariably meant I would experience those feelings again, which was a complete mindfuck.

The second week of December, during a therapy session with Caroline, I talked about how everything seemed to be getting worse.

"Call WCPR to see if there is any way you can get into a sooner retreat. Just give it a try. Miles told you to call him if you needed anything, right? What can it hurt?"

I paused to consider and immediately the berating thoughts surfaced. *What kind of captain asks for a spot in front of someone else? The captain goes down with the ship. The captain eats last, showers last, and leaves the building on fire last.*

I'd already abandoned my crew at BFD. How could I ask to step in front of someone else?

"Just see if a spot has opened up," she said. "I know you don't ask for help. Just try. Please."

For two days I ruminated. A fierce argument broke out inside my head whether to continue to be the stoic captain who handles everything alone or to take the risk and ask for help. I knew something had to change on this path of hopelessness I insisted on staying on. I decided Caroline was right . . . it wouldn't hurt to ask. Even talking to Miles might help. It had the first time, and he said to call if I needed anything.

I dialed his number. The phone rang and rang. Finally, someone picked up, and the person on the other line sounded completely irritated.

"Yeah."

"Is this Miles Pond?"

"Yeah."

"Hi . . . uh . . . this is Christy Warren. I talked to you last month about attending WCPR."

"Yeah."

"Well, um . . . ah . . . .I . . . I was wondering if you happen to have anything sooner. I'm drowning."

"Nope. Sorry. You're just going to have to suck it up until March."

"Ok . . . um . . . thanks."

He hung up without a goodbye or see you in a few months.

Fuck that fucking fuck. He said to call if I needed anything and now he is telling me to suck it up? What a dick! This is what happens when I ask for help. This is why I don't ask for help.

Tears rolled down my face. I willed the tears to stop. Like flipping a switch, I shut down the little tantrum in my head. I was done. WCPR advertised they understood and they were going to help and support me—and this stupid fuck treated me like this?

I was done. No more tears from me. No more trying to open up. Whatever soft pieces remained of me were crushed so quickly and fully, only fire and hardness endured. I believed with my entire being that healing was hopeless. I worried Lisa would leave me, but I could not shut off the noise in my head. I sank deeper into quicksand.

"When did mom say she's showing up?" I asked my brother, after arriving at his house on Christmas Day.

Every Christmas morning, my brother and his wife, the girls (he had two of them now), me, and my mom waited until we were all together to open presents. Lisa stayed home because all that activity and people were too much for her, though she did sometimes come over for Christmas dinner.

My brother met my gaze. "Well, she said she'd be here at noon."

It was already noon.

I helped myself to a cup of coffee and watched the girls bounce around the room, jittering with controlled anticipation of opening the giant avalanche of gifts that flowed from under the Christmas tree.

Kat couldn't stand it anymore and bellowed loud enough so everyone could hear. "When is Grandma going to get here?"

Grandma arrived an hour later, bringing with her all the usual reasons for being late. She'd been late my entire life. I was so used to it, I wasn't even fazed. I just felt bad for the girls.

The day after Christmas, motivated to get out of the house, I had a free afternoon and decided to see a movie by myself. I wouldn't dwell on the past or the future. I would only think of right now.

I walked into the theater, found a seat, and shut my phone off. Sitting in the dark, focusing on the movie, I felt some peace.

I walked out of the theater with my spirits lifted. As I walked out, I turned my phone back on and saw I had a missed call from a Santa Rosa number.

Frowning, already knowing who it was, I listened to the message. "This is Miles Pond. Call me back."

Why? So, you can make me feel like a worthless pile of shit again? No thank you.

As I exited the theater complex's main doors, I ran into someone who I worshipped as a kid—my former summer camp counselor at Caritas Creek. I hadn't seen her in twenty years. She'd always filled me with hope when things were shitty back home. I had felt valued and that I mattered when I was around her.

She gave me a giant hug. We talked until she needed to get inside for the movie she was going to see. Reconnecting with her brought back memories, which served up another dose of positivity on the heels of the movie.

It was the best I'd felt in a while. When I got home and told Lisa Miles had called, her face expressed happiness.

"Well, did you call him back?"

"Hell, no. Fuck that guy. He isn't going to make me feel like a piece of shit again."

"Please call him," she said. "Just see what he says."

"I'll think about it." About thirty minutes later, my phone rang again. Santa Rosa again. Reluctantly, I answered.

"This is Miles Pond. I'm glad you answered because I was about to go onto the next person. I got a spot for you. Can you be there January fourth?"

"Yes! Oh my God, thank you."

"Yeah, you sounded pretty bad."

The anger I'd been harboring toward Miles washed away in an instant. The weight I'd been carrying like an immense boulder, crushing me every day, lifted off of my body. I didn't know if I would have made it until March.

The lightness I felt lasted approximately two hours because that afternoon, a letter landed in my mailbox from ACS.

After careful consideration of all available information, we are denying liability for your claim of injury. Workers' compensation benefits are being denied because we have insufficient factual and medical evidence to show your claimed injury is work-related. In addition, your Panel Qualified Medical Examination is scheduled after our 90th-day decision date.

As pissed as I was, my examiner from ACS had told me to expect this letter. She also said if the QME decided my injury was work-related, they would notify me that they accepted my claim. So, the soonest my claim could be accepted was February 19, five months after I went off work.

Thank God I didn't have a family to support and didn't live paycheck to paycheck. Thank God I had savings. If I got another job, my workers' comp claim would automatically be thrown in the trash. I was paying $310 a week to see therapists. I'd just paid $3,000 to attend a retreat that I hoped would right this sinking ship. Imagine having a broken leg and waiting five months to see a doctor.

I began to think the folks who ran workers' comp were actually trying to kill me. If I killed myself, they wouldn't have to spend another dime.

CHAPTER TWENTY-FOUR

I lived the rest of December day by day, sometimes hour by hour. Then New Year's Eve 2014 landed. My plans were to spend the night at my friends Julie and Ray's house. They were having a small party with a handful of my great friends.

The constant insanity in my head still hadn't let up. *I am tired of shitty calls playing over and over*, I thought as I drove to Julie and Ray's. *I am tired of the anxiety. I am tired of my worthless life and ending up a horrible failure.*

After a forty-five-minute drive, I pulled up to the house and parked in front. Daylight still hung around, but the sun had started its disappearing act. Julie and Ray's fantastic blow-up Christmas decorations sat deflated and sagged over to one side on their lawn, laying on the ground.

I am going to get shit-faced tonight. I am going to shut it down. A wave of giddiness rolled through me. With my sleeping bag and an overnight backpack, I walked up the driveway and down the path to their front door. I paused at the deflated decorations as I knocked on the door. Santa and his elves looked like they'd been the victims of a drive-by shooting.

I played ice hockey with all of these friends, and we'd become close. We traveled together and went out together. I always felt safe with them and knew their love and friendship was unconditional.

Julie and Ray's two large dogs greeted me at the door as soon as Julie opened it.

"There is beer in the garage," Julie said, by way of welcoming me, "but you have to get it yourself."

The dogs clogged the hallway to the garage entrance, demanding belly rubs and ear scratches. I promised them I would be back as soon as I got a beer.

The first cold beer went down quickly. So did the second. The traditional New Year's Eve football game was on, but I sat on the couch and stared right through the TV. The third beer, thirty minutes after I arrived, went down nice, too.

With each beer I felt happier. The buzz was nice, but what I was really excited about was the silence melting into my head. It was like being in a long line at Disneyland and finally getting near the front.

"Let's play Cards Against Humanity," Julie's brother Matt said.

I sat down at the small kitchen table, along with my friend Amanda, Matt and his wife Cathie, Julie's sister, Monica, and a few other friends, but quickly got back up. "Wait just one minute, I need another beer."

"Forget the beer," Matt said, "I will make you a drink."

I sat back down and soon Matt handed me a drink in a tall milk glass. I threw the first one back like a person lost in the desert would first drink water, except I didn't spill it down the front of me. Yet. Matt made me another drink . . . and then another . . . and another.

As we played, I lost every round. I sat at the table, unable to figure out why I always got creamed at Cards Against Humanity. It didn't matter because around the fourth cocktail, everything went dark.

I vaguely remember the countdown and everyone yelling, "Happy New Year!"

The next thing I knew, I was kneeling on the bathroom floor, my arms draped around a porcelain toilet. My head was resting on my right arm. A large piece of drool hung from my lips.

Cathie handed me a towel to wipe my face.

"I'm so sorry," I mumbled.

"It's okay, Christy."

"I'm so sorry," I said again. My stomach contracted again, spewing out my insides. Tears squeezed out of my eyes, and my chest heaved to catch my breath.

The lights and sounds shut down again. Everything disappeared.

My eyes slowly blinked open and took a few minutes to focus. I was on the floor, seeing the room from a new perspective. The sun had come up, and I found myself alone in a small room, which appeared to be the place in Julie and Ray's house that I had planned to sleep in. I was on carpet, so I knew I was not in the bathroom anymore.

I was half on/half off an air mattress and a quarter in/three-quarters out of my sleeping bag. My clothes were soaking wet. I was grateful to discover it was water. I was wearing the same clothes from last night. My head felt like a split piece of wood, and my tongue had thickened overnight and produced its own cotton crop. Yet I had not felt this level of relief in a long time. My head had finally shut off for almost six hours. No nightmares, no waking up in a panic, screaming and frustrated. Everything had just disappeared for six glorious hours. The wonderfulness of shutting down the shitshow in my brain outweighed the physical misery of an epic hangover or the embarrassment of vomiting.

Dousing my brain in alcohol had stopped me from having to feel anything. Lately, the ghosts kept chasing and haunting me, so I did not dare stop moving. Last night, the ghosts had been stripped of their haunting powers.

Even though my body felt as if a large garbage truck had run over it, I couldn't remember how long it had been since I'd been this joyful. The silent darkness of blacking out, followed by the dull fog overtaking my body, gave me a brief reprieve from the noise and panic.

On New Year's Day, deflated and quiet, I finally got a little rest.

CHAPTER TWENTY-FIVE

Three days later, the morning of Sunday, January 4, 2015, time moved so slowly I watched and felt the second hand tick every single second. I'd look at the clock, and then look back again, and the minute hand hadn't moved. I was finally leaving for the retreat! I couldn't wait to find some peace, but at the same time, my body shook with fear. The payoff could be significant, but the cost could be insurmountable. What if they discovered my inherent weakness? What if they confirmed how defective I was?

The gravity of the process and the possible complications almost overwhelmed me to where I thought, *Maybe it'd be better to live with the pain.*

I packed my clothes using my work duffle bag. I stared at it now and wondered what everyone would think of it. After a few minutes, I moved everything into a suitcase. *No, that will make me look stupid. One whole suitcase for five days of sitting around?* I put my clothes back in the duffle bag.

The retreat was being held in the mountains of Northern California, about a one-hour drive from my house. Trees, bushes, and nature lined both sides of the narrow drive off the main road. As Lisa drove us up the long, steep driveway to the retreat, my shoulders tensed up to where they were almost touching my ears. My lips were mashed so tightly together, it was as if they'd sealed themselves so nothing would leak out. I wore my biggest and best "I don't give a fuck" look and crossed my arms over my chest in defiance.

Coming here is a total mistake. I don't think I can do this. This place is dumb, and I am so uncomfortable. I would much prefer running into a burning building than walk into this place. If Lisa wasn't the one driving, I'd have turned around and gone back home.

At the top of the driveway sat a big, dark-brown, three-story house. A chubby, gray-haired guy came out with a warm smile on his face and introduced himself as Tracy.

I immediately thought, *I am in the wrong place. This guy looks like he would rather sit and eat doughnuts than bust a door down.* I was afraid I had become and maybe always been, a token woman firefighter, not the real deal.

Tracy welcomed us and showed us around. The dining and day room were inside the front door. We walked into the large commercial size kitchen.

Tracy said, "Here is the kitchen. If there is anything you want or need, just ask and we will make it happen."

I thought, *What the fuck? This is stupid. It's just a fucking kitchen.*

He would say something positive, and I'd say "okay" out loud, but my internal reaction to everything was, *Whatever.*

After the tour, I walked back out to the car to get my duffle bag and sleeping bag.

Lisa started crying and said to me, "It is so hard for me to leave you here."

I was shocked. I figured she would be happy to get rid of me and all my craziness for a week. I started crying, too. When I turned to leave, Tracy watched us with soft, kind eyes.

"Don't worry," he said to Lisa. "We'll take good care of her. We won't let her out of our sight."

A blanket of safety had been thrown over me. He was okay with the mess of my life. And he was also okay I had prepared myself for some members of the organization to be homophobic. Now I could relax and not dance around that important part of my life.

After watching Lisa's car head down the driveway until it disappeared around the corner, I walked back inside the building.

Tracy said, "Luke is ready for you to sign in and handle your payment. He's in the office straight ahead."

I walked into the office, and Luke introduced himself. He was the real deal . . . the kind of guy I admired. Sturdy, fit, and smart, he had once been army special-forces and a long-time cop. He was the very person I desperately needed to tell me I was worthy, even though I was falling apart.

And of course, about thirty seconds after I sat down, I started crying.

Luke, the badass, looked me straight in the eyes and said, "Well, let me tell you the deal. Your job this week is to cry through three-thousand dollars worth of Kleenex." I signed all the paperwork and handed over my check for the retreat fee of $3,000.

A small smile emerged on my face, even as my tears continued. "Thank you," I said.

I walked out of that office and back to my chair I had chosen in the corner. Luke and Tracy gave me hope and made me feel safe. They liked me and wanted me to be there.

The volunteer staff of WCPR included two clinicians, five to fifteen peers, and a chaplain. The clinicians were culturally competent, meaning they specialized in treating first responders and primarily only saw first responders and their families. The peers were all first responders who had been through the WCPR retreat as a client or were experts in peer support. All the peers were in different stages of their recovery.

Five tables filled half of the large room. Seven of us clients were instructed to sit around a specific table. The remaining tables were for the peers, clinicians, and the cook. They covered the round tables with brown, vinyl tablecloths. A box of Kleenex and hand sanitizer made up the centerpiece. A large TV screen was affixed to the wall above the mantel of a no-longer-used fireplace. The other half of the room had two couches and sofa chairs set up in a square, just like a living room. Large windows lined this large room and had a view over and through large pine and oak trees. A peaceful lake made up the distant view. But on this first day of the retreat, I never noticed the view. I could barely look past my own feet.

The first client I encountered after sitting down at the table was Madison. Immediately, the judgments began.

Madison was slim and appeared to weigh very little. She was a cop. *Typical woman who has no business being a cop*, I thought. She was obviously here because she couldn't handle the job. She was pretty, wore makeup, and very feminine clothes.

Terry had a heavy, southern accent and smoked. *No doubt this guy hates gays. I am sure he doesn't think women should be cops or firefighters.*

Garrett was a badass motherfucker. Another cop. He was big and tall and strong. Tattoos covered his arms and legs. His hair was slicked back, and he wore a black T-shirt that said something angry. Thank God for Garrett.

Macy looked just like me. Void of any makeup, she wore jeans and a T-shirt, and had super-short hair. *Great. Just great. She's probably angry and bossy and will want to talk about gay crap the whole time.*

The only other firefighter client, Greg, appeared sad and

ruined. He walked with his head down and his mouth appeared as if he had both edges surgically pulled down. Greg was just a regular guy.

Tom talked like he had gravel in his throat. He was built thick as an old-growth redwood tree. Even his fingers were like plump sausages, and they were easy to see because he couldn't talk without waving his hands around. His body parts continued to move in nervous tics, and his leg never stopped bouncing. He spun around like a top, so fast that it felt like I'd never get a look at what was painted on the sides.

I would later figure out my relentlessly harsh judgment of people had to do with my incessant comparison of myself to others. I tended to identify with whatever group I was with—so I preferred to surround myself with powerful people, a projection of who I desperately wanted to be. I had to make a declaration of who was strong because I reasoned if I walked with the strong, I, too, would be strong and valuable. If I walked with weakness, then my fate was sealed. I would be worthless. I yearned for the day when comparing myself to others was no longer instinctual, no longer the first step I took when I met someone new.

But for now, the only people in my peer group who would get even a modicum of respect from me would be the strong ones—Luke and Garrett.

The peers started off with introductions and immediately I knew I was in the right place. These were fourteen people who had been through the same thing as me. They were all here for the same reasons I was here, and they were all listening and attentive.

Maybe I am not the only one. I softened slightly.

After introductions, it was time for dinner.

Prior to the retreat, I had worried about what I would eat. I had an inherent negative reaction to gluten. But despite the prior email requests to inform them of food allergies, I didn't specify anything.

However, when I had first arrived, the cook, Big Joe, had asked everyone again about food allergies, with a demeanor indicating he would kick anyone's ass who lied. So I quietly and casually informed him I couldn't eat gluten. But I didn't expect him to adjust to my eating issues.

When we walked into the kitchen for that first dinner, there sat a large pan of homemade macaroni and cheese. Big Joe tapped me on the shoulder and pointed away from the other food. A steaming hot dish of gluten-free macaroni and cheese sat on the counter.

It had been years since I'd been able to eat mac n' cheese. I was so touched. This was an intimate gift, a small gesture that was monumental to me. Someone had taken the time to do something extra for me. My heart swelled in gratitude for Big Joe's actions.

After dinner, as my journal stated, "We shared a bunch of shit." We partnered up and asked each other a set of questions about why were we there, why now, and what would be the first thing we'd notice when we were better.

When we finished interviewing each other, we introduced who we just interviewed to the group. All twenty-four people at the retreat (peers, clinicians, chaplain, and clients) sat around, focused on us. Everyone listened attentively. Luke would often step in and ask more questions about our answers.

In the end, we learned all seven of us were fucked up. We all had the same symptoms: anxiety, depression, isolation, nightmares, anger, and suicidal feelings.

I admitted to them how weak I was, and although I found solace that they were going through the same thing, I still clung onto the belief it shouldn't be happening to me.

After the evening activities ended, I had no desire to talk, so I headed for bed. I found a little piece of paper left on my pillow with a quote that read, "Life begins at the end of your comfort zone."

That's for fucking sure.

CHAPTER TWENTY-SIX

Despite watching the ceiling, walls, and the lamp all night, I felt lighter in the morning than I had the previous night. As I walked downstairs from the bedrooms to the table room/ living room area, the smell of bacon improved my mood even more.

Every peer I walked by wore a smile on their face, said, "Good morning" and asked how I had slept. They were welcoming. And I didn't have to cook or clean up. All I had to do was eat.

First responders who went to WCPR as clients struggled with having someone else clean up after them. Being taken care of in this manner is foreign. Many of us grew up having to take care of ourselves or younger siblings or even our parents. When we became professional rescuers, we put the needs of an entire city before our own.

It was Monday, technically Day Two, but our first full day at the retreat. We began with a morning check-in, where each person talked about how they were doing and any new insights gained or triggers they experienced.

As soon as the first person started talking, my tears fell for the hundredth time, for no reason. I leaned over so my forehead rested on the table. My tears fell onto the floor directly under my face.

Mark, a clinician, stopped the conversation and spoke to me

with a tender voice. "Hey Christy, what's going on?"

What? Are you talking to me? Someone cares enough to stop everything and check on me? I felt caught. I'd been hoping my tears wouldn't draw attention. I wanted to be cared for but the protective part of me begged for him to move on. I paused and looked around, as if he might have been addressing someone else.

"Yes, you Christy. Tell us what the tears are about."

Warmth seeped into my chest, and my shoulders softened a little. "I really don't know, exactly," I said slowly. "But you know when you have to go pee for a long time and you're holding it and doing okay, but then the closer you get to the bathroom, the harder it is to hold? Well, this feels just like that. I think I've been holding back tears for forty-four years and I'm finally someplace where I can let it go."

Mark smiled. "Well, you are in the right place. I'm glad you are here."

"Thanks," I said—but I also said to myself, *How in the hell can you be glad I am here when you don't even know me?*

After check-in, they sent us to a room to take some psych tests. They asked questions like, "Have you ever thought of suicide? Have you ever almost lost your life at work?"

Immediately, the man I forgot to finish looking for at 2025 Oregon Street burst into my awareness. I reactively threw my pencil down and started rubbing my hands on my thighs. I wanted out of that room.

Garrett looked directly at me and said, "Just keep writing."

I picked the pencil back up and kept at it. *No way in hell am I going to talk about this. Then everyone will know for sure what a terrible captain I am, and I never really belonged in the fire service.*

In the afternoon, we went through a series of interviews by two peers who dug deeper into our family and personal histories.

I got the two CHP officers, Larry and Barb. Barb was a tall, sturdy woman with an intense focus. She wore dark-blue cotton pants, a sweatshirt, and comfortable shoes. She sat in front of me and asked basic questions, and then follow-up questions based on the intake form and phone interviews I'd done before coming.

"How old were you when your parents divorced?"

"How much alcohol did your mom drink?"

"How often did she drive drunk with you in the car?"

"What kind of drugs did your stepfather do? Your mom?"

"Did your mom say anything when she walked in on it but never put a stop to it?"

"How old were you when your brother left to live with your dad?"

"How old were you when you went to live with your grandmother?"

I answered her questions with complete honesty, except for the fire with the limp, ashen, dead guy I had failed.

As usual, I took every chance to belittle myself. In the middle of yet another self-disparaging answer, Barb interrupted me.

"When are you going to give yourself the very same grace you give others?"

Her words and eyes bored through me. She had hit me with a *Star Trek* phaser set for stun.

My lips and jaw tightened. I had no answer. All I could do was stare back at her.

That evening, we gathered for our first session in the Rubber Room. The Rubber Room was a large open room with ceilings about twenty feet high. Floor-to-ceiling windows lined one side of the room with the nature view outside. Couches and big comfortable chairs lined the perimeter, making an oval shape.

The debriefing happened in this room. Here we talked about events we had told no one about. The cops shared about being shot, having to shoot someone, or having their partner shot and killed beside them. Firefighters and paramedics talked about not being able to save the lives of kids. Dispatchers spoke about listening to screams coming from the other end of the phone line and not being able to do anything about it. We shared stories from our childhoods. We shared whatever trauma we had experienced that continued to hold us underwater.

The first part of the "debriefing" was the fact stage. They wanted us to talk about the facts of our critical incident that brought us there. The seven of us plus two clinicians, a chaplain, and the two peers, Barb and Luke, sat in circle. The clients migrated to the ends of the couches, each clutching a pillow . . . except for Tom. He regularly moved between sitting and standing.

Garrett went first. He chose a childhood incident to talk about. An older neighbor kid had sexually abused the young and naive Garrett. Garrett told us how this older kid used attention and treats to manipulate him into performing sexual acts. His voice shook, but he spoke with determination and pure authenticity. The older kid started off with simple treats in exchange for small sexual deeds. Then the treats became more significant and so did the acts. Garrett craved the attention, but over time it was confusing, and he was too far in. The older kid warned Garrett that if he told anyone, he would get in serious trouble. The trap was laid, and he didn't know how to get out.

I talked about an innocuous fire in a three-story apartment building on Dwight Street where I was concerned for the safety of my crew and myself. The paralyzing shame of my performance, or lack thereof, on the Oregon Street fire, bounded that incident in the back of my throat. I couldn't share it with the group, so instead I chose another incident and made it sound as dramatic as possible, worried that if I didn't talk about something heavy, they would call me on it and dig until they found something heavy. The dead guy from the Oregon Street fire lay so close to the surface they would surely find him if they dug at all, and I couldn't have that.

Madison told stories of what she went through as a police officer. Listening to her story, I realized this lady was so much tougher than I gave her credit for.

The southern guy I thought was a redneck hick? He was a hick, but he was also an amazing, loving, and kind man. His son was gay, and this dad couldn't be prouder.

Meanwhile, Macy, the woman who reminded me of myself, was just a regular person living her life—a person who believed you should work hard and earn respect, not demand it.

I had made ridiculous snap judgments of these people, the very thing I was always afraid of people doing to me. Spending the day sharing some of our hardest secrets garnered respect for everyone in my group. Just after a single sharing session, I felt a kinship with my group based on empathy and respect.

We finished in the Rubber Room around 10:00 p.m., and despite the darkness, all of us went for a walk. Garrett and I brought up the rear.

I placed a gentle hand on Garrett's arm and said, "The thing that happened to you? Well, the same thing happened to me. So, I understand."

Garrett said nothing, but I knew he'd heard me. I just wanted him to know he was not alone. I had shoved that subject to the very bottom of the box, so I'd never known how it had affected me.

Worried Garrett might try to continue the conversation, I moved on quickly. "Wow, look at those stars," I said. "Beautiful, aren't they?"

The next morning, after not sleeping for shit, I got up early, my body needing to move. I had to run hard. Not for exercise but because my insides were ready to blow out of my skin. I hated running in the morning, but the alternative of not going was worse.

Megan, a peer, waited downstairs for anyone who wanted to go for a run. She was fit and dressed in fine running apparel. I wore what I'd slept in—some shitty T-shirt with holes in the armpits and a pair of BFD mesh shorts.

We took off down the steep driveway and onto the road not much wider than the driveway. Blackberry bushes, oak trees, and ferns lined both sides of the road. We ran past a few dirt driveways, which led to houses tucked behind the forestry. The cool morning air soothed my skin, but my lungs burned, and my muscles ached. I used to be in good shape, but I hadn't worked out in three months other than my anxiety runs. Still, I had to keep up with Megan, so she wouldn't think, "What kind of loser firefighter is Christy? She can't run for shit. How in the hell can she be a firefighter if she can't even run?"

I fell into the same pattern I always did, either judging or worried about being judged. Every step, I struggled to keep up.

We finally arrived back at the bottom of the steep, long hill that led to the retreat house. Everything in my body burned and cramped. I had to win this run. If I didn't, I'd be outed as the token worthless woman firefighter. I put my head down and demanded my leg muscles to move faster.

I made it to the top—behind Megan. I'd failed. I was disgusted with myself. I couldn't even look Megan in the eyes.

Later, during that morning's check-in, when Megan took her turn, she said, "The day started off with a beautiful morning run with Christy. We saw the sunrise and the light filtered through the trees. It was beautiful."

I then realized that I'd run a race that no one else had entered. As usual.

Everything was a competition for me. If someone talked

about having to wear a mouthguard at night, I told them how I have bitten through two of them—the extra thick ones. If someone said they broke their leg once, I said I have broken both of my legs. I had to be the best. I had to win. It was all or nothing.

As soon as my turn came for check-in, I started crying again. These endless tears just kept coming. I began to wonder if I would ever stop crying.

I had spent my whole life being angry to cover the despair of growing up invisible, alone, and unloved. Anger and invulnerability equaled survival.

But here at the retreat, the anger was replaced by something else. I was realizing it was time to stop escaping or trying to pretend I was okay or tough.

After breakfast and check-in, our butts remained in our chairs, waiting for the first video to start. It was a thirty-minute video about police suicide. The cop on the screen told us, in detail, about how he had put a gun in his mouth and almost pulled the trigger. His wife stopped him in time. Another wife, a mother, and a father talked about the downward spiral their loved ones fell into until they hit the bottom and killed themselves. Some experts talked about the effects of the job and how it could lead to suicide.

Suddenly, Terry got out of his chair and ran out the room. A peer immediately followed him.

I was stunned, but Luke offered some context for us. "That cop who talks about how he almost killed himself is a Memphis cop. So, you can imagine how Terry feels watching that. He was a Memphis cop."

After about ten minutes, Terry slowly walked back in, his face red and wet. He shook his head and whimpered, "So many suicides. So many of my friends have killed themselves. So many I have tried to help."

During the day, they asked us to write down our "critical incidents." I started to list mine. I filled an entire 8.5 x 11 piece of paper, even writing outside the margins, until I needed a second piece. Seeing the number of calls listed instilled the magnitude of just how much misery, death, trauma, and sorrow I'd witnessed and been a part of. A small flash of reason darted through my brain. *I really need to stop telling myself what a failure I am for being affected by all I have witnessed.*

After dinner, our group made the outdoor walk from the main house, across the grounds, and slowly plodded up, stair by stair, into the Rubber Room. Everyone took their same seat and grabbed their same pillow. We began the "feelings" stage of our critical incident.

Sitting on my end of the couch clutching my pillow, I felt calm and comfortable. When my turn came, I talked more about the fire on Dwight Street—the dilemma I'd faced there, and my fear of putting my crew in danger.

After I finished sharing, no one said anything. Clinician Dian thanked me, and we moved on to Garrett. I felt relief and disappointment. Telling that story as my critical incident, I was full of shit. Everything I'd said about the fire was true, but everyone had gotten out of the building safely. It wasn't an incident that had stayed with me; it wasn't a call that had needed to go into the box.

While I perseverated, Garrett talked about how being molested made him feel rotted and broken inside. He had spent his whole life desperately keeping the incident hidden from his being, from everyone, so they wouldn't find out how truly rancid and undeserving he was. He'd built an impenetrable suit of armor reinforced with confidence. By being the guy who rescued everyone else, no one would think to glance at his insides.

I sat there, clutching my pillow. As Garrett continued, my insides grabbed onto his words. *Holy shit, this is my story.*

Something started to build inside me, like a water pump turning on and the water starts to bubble up. I felt it in the deepest part of me I didn't know existed. The more Garrett talked, the faster the pump worked. It quickly became a fire hydrant that had been sheared off by an out-of-control car. My ribbon spun out of control.

I have to get out of here. I'm going to blow. But it's Garrett's turn. I will be an asshole if I leave, interrupting Garrett's story. I have to get out of here.

With no control over my body, I lurched up and forward for the door. I accelerated with each step, like I was running for my life. I ran out the front door and down the steps. I hit the pavement of the parking area and kept running. I ran about thirty feet when the tall, strong CHP lady caught me. Then I blew. I was the fire hydrant, sobbing like I'd never sobbed before.

Barb put her arms around me. She stood much taller than me, so my wailing face fit right up against the front of her shoulder. My crying came from somewhere inside my core. My legs and body went limp. Barb held me up in her hug and quietly told me to breathe.

Once I stopped crying and could breathe again, we walked back up the stairs into the Rubber Room. I sat back down in my spot and grabbed a pillow. Mark asked me to tell to the group what had happened to me.

"It's Garrett's turn," I said. "I will go after he is done. It was extraordinarily rude of me to interrupt him," I said. "I'm very sorry."

But Mark and the group were unyielding. I had to talk immediately.

I wiped the snot off my face and said, "What happened to

Garrett happened to me, but it was my stepbrother. I have also built armor so no one can see how rotten and defective I am inside cuz if your own mother doesn't love you, then you must not be lovable. If your dad complains about what a burden you are to pick up every other weekend, you are not worthy. If you have sex with your older stepbrother when you are six, you are pretty disgusting. If the secret got out of who I was or what I had done, I'd be ruined."

I told the group my story—my real story—and no one judged me. Peers I respected learned the truth about me and they stayed, listening and caring. At that moment, I could say I was worthy. I deserved love and happiness. It was the first time I had ever thought that . . . and meant it.

Wednesday morning I was exhausted, like the anesthesia had just worn off from a long and miserable surgery. My stomach hurt. My eyes were swollen. I had zero desire to get out of bed. But I did. I had to.

Slowly, one by one, the empty chairs filled in around the table downstairs after breakfast. We all looked like crap.

Again, as soon as check-in began, I started to cry. I sat there with tears running down my face until my turn to talk arrived. I shut the flood down long enough for me to share. After check-in, we headed back to the Rubber Room to finish our debriefing.

That night, I slept from midnight to 3:00 a.m. I finally got up once the morning sunlight filtered through the trees into our room. I stumbled to the bathroom and saw myself in the mirror. I looked like shit again.

Many peers asked how I was doing, and I answered honestly, "I'm not sure. I'm still trying to figure it out." I felt like a large ball of knotted rope had been removed from the inside of me.

But the gaping open hole left me feeling exposed.

I cried again during the entire check-in.

✒

Thursday was Day Four and Family Day in the Rubber Room, where we talked about our childhoods and our families.

Everyone in my group, like me, had a craptacular childhood. I had been protecting this great secret of how I was raised, when so many others held onto this same secret that grew into a garden of shame. Macy, who reminded me of myself, had a mother just like mine.

On the last morning, I cried again during check-in, as I had every morning since arriving. But this time I noticed something different. My head wasn't in my hands. I sat up straight. I no longer hid my tears with my head down.

I wanted to have all my new fucked-up friends sign the Kleenex box I'd been relying on, so I could take it home with me as a reminder. I passed the Kleenex box and a black Sharpie around the table. Terry, Madison, Tom, Garrett, Macy, and Greg passed it around and signed it.

As we finished up, I looked out the window, and I saw Lisa's car making the long uphill drive to the house. My eyes, ears, brain, heart, shoulders, stomach, and toes locked onto her car. Something good exploded in me. I couldn't wait to get to her. I sat like an Olympic runner at the starting blocks of the gold medal race.

After the last person stopped talking, the starting gun went off and I ran to the parking lot. Lisa sat in her car, reading. I banged on the window, and she got out of the car, slightly startled. I put my arms around her and wouldn't let go, thinking, *I'm here, I get it, I'm alive, we are going to make it, I am going to make it.* I must have kissed her face fifty times.

When I finally stopped and turned around, my entire group was in a semicircle behind us. They reached out to her for hugs and handshakes. An amazing feeling of pride and love spread all over me until I finally understood the sentiment behind having a full heart. My heart was full.

On the way home, I talked and talked and cried and cried. Lisa cried too. I couldn't stop talking about the amazing people I met and how much I'd learned and how I wasn't the only one with this PTSD bullshit. I even felt a little bit good about myself.

WCPR saved my life. I finally understood what I was going through, and I understood I was not alone. So many tough cops and firefighters had PTSD. WCPR helped me to see PTSD didn't mean I was a failure. It didn't mean I wasn't enough. It didn't mean I was a bad firefighter. Having PTSD meant I had seen so much trauma, it caused a physical injury to my brain.

Those first few days after I came home, I could see the relief Lisa finally experienced. The magnitude of her relief equalled if I'd been in a horrible car accident, where she'd been in the surgery waiting room for hours, until finally the doctor came out and told her I was going to live.

I felt like I'd been given a second chance.

PART III

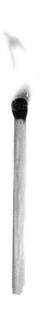

CHAPTER TWENTY-SEVEN

My first day home from the retreat, I carried a laundry basket full of dirty clothes out to the garage. Light on my feet, I was still buoyed by the experience.

I opened the front-loading washing machine door—and the hole came alive to suck me in. My vision tunneled inside as my entire body recoiled. The ribbon came out of nowhere. The dark opening exposed what I had done at the retreat. My stomach twisted and my chest hurt.

I ruined everything. I told a bunch of people my secrets. I opened myself up like a cracked-open pomegranate—all the little pieces inside of me—exposed. I made myself vulnerable and my weaknesses visible to everyone. I swore I wouldn't ask anyone for help. Now I've broken my vow. What was I thinking?

The WCPR staff knew refusing to ask for help was a tendency among first responders. They'd addressed how much we struggled to make the call for help by referring to it as "picking up the five-hundred-pound phone."

The next day, I actually thought about picking up that five-hundred-pound phone. A handful of times throughout the day, I even dialed my cell phone—but never pressed the "send" button.

I spent most of the day at war with myself. *Do I trust people from WCPR? The ones who said to pick up the phone and someone will be there for me? What if they aren't? It will prove I'm not worthy of anyone's help.*

But I needed help. I needed help to get back to living. *If I don't,* I thought, *why would Lisa stick around?*

So, finally, I took a deep breath and an enormous risk. I picked up that five-hundred-pound phone, dialed the number, and hit "send." I called Barb, and I shared my sudden descent into despair after having felt so good for a few days.

She said to me, "Give yourself the same grace that you give others. Write out your values. Work to change the dialogue in your head. Stop and ask yourself, "What is really going on?""

These were the exact words I needed to hear. I opened my journal I had started while at the retreat and wrote everything I was afraid of or felt helpless about. I even wrote something positive about myself.

I was learning that confronting my true feelings and not berating myself for them was the work I needed to do to get better. Self-compassion was the antidote to shame. For me to stop minimizing everything I'd been through and to have this self-compassion was going to take a village.

When I returned to Caroline's office for EMDR therapy after the retreat, everything I learned and gained at WCPR poured out of me.

The montage of calls, which played over and over in my head always began with the same call, and then played in the same order. We decided to tackle these calls again. She handed me the two hand buzzers to begin EMDR.

They lightly buzzed back and forth, left hand . . . right hand . . . left hand . . . right hand. I closed my eyes and Caroline asked me what I could see.

"It is night out. I am kneeling on the ground at the heads of a husband and wife who were ejected from the front windshield. They are lying next to each other." I felt the gravel I was kneeling in. I heard the *whoosh* and saw the blur of cars flying by in my peripheral vision along the freeway. I felt the rush of air as they drove by. I saw the flood of light coming from our ambulance. I felt the laryngoscope handle in my hand. I saw the green bag lying open, displaying medical supplies to maintain a person's airway.

Holy shit—this EMDR thing is finally working. I felt like I was actually there on the side of the freeway in the dark. Before, the memory had existed as a one-dimensional photo. Now the memory had come alive, and I was there.

"What kind of emotion are you feeling?"

"I'm frustrated. Who in the hell am I supposed to intubate first?"

"What do you think about yourself right now?"

"I feel helpless. No matter what choice I make, someone is going to lose."

"What would you like to think about yourself?"

"That I am doing the best I can, and it's just a shitty situation. That the situation I'm in is not a reflection on me not being able to do the right thing."

As soon as we were done for the day, the haunting scene faded. The memory remained, but it no longer felt like a hammer constantly banging at my head.

My work at WCPR had made all the difference. I was so shut down before that I would let nothing in and nothing out. Now there was a crack in my armor, and EMDR was able to open it wider.

The problem with cracks, though, is that they let light in— but they also allow access to the dark, tangled mess inside of you.

CHAPTER TWENTY-EIGHT

Friday evening of Martin Luther King Jr. weekend, I heaved my bulky hockey bag into the trunk of my car. I threw my sticks in the back seat and shook my head at the countless black marks on the back seat of my gray Acura. I grabbed my plethora of water bottles, kissed Lisa goodbye, and headed out the door.

Hockey has always been the best antidepressant for me. When I am on the ice, I think of nothing else except chasing that small black hunk of vulcanized rubber. If I arrive at the ice rink in a foul mood, I always leave in a good mood. Not only is it the game but also the people I play with.

I was particularly excited about this tournament, which the San Jose Sharks hosted every year on MLK weekend, because so many of my friends would be there.

I pulled out onto the freeway and made my way toward San Jose. About fifteen minutes into my drive, I passed a big green sign on the right side of the freeway that read, "Ken Youngstrom Memorial Freeway." My brain flashed to a photo of the scene where he was killed. A good friend of mine was one of the first responders to arrive on scene, and he'd described to me every detail of what had happened to Ken Youngstrom. My body tensed at the memory.

I kept driving. Farther down the freeway, fifteen minutes later, the same green sign, this time with another CHP officer's name on it, grabbed my eye. Now my brain flashed to visual of the husband and wife who were ejected out of the windshield of their car.

Another twenty minutes down the road, another green sign with another CHP officer's name on it. This time my brain flashed to Lakeville Road in Vallejo, 1996. I was a paramedic working on the ambulance in Vallejo. A pickup truck had rolled several times in the middle of the night, on a sparsely traveled road. When we arrived on scene, a CHP car had its spotlight directly on a twenty-something-year-old kid lying on his back, his arms and legs contorted into positions no alive human body could achieve. His face looked like someone had taken a baseball bat to it.

As I continued to drive down the freeway toward San Jose, this scene played over and over in my mind, until my eyes saw yet another memorial sign and another CHP call—two guys pushing their broken-down car on the Carquinez Bridge were crushed when a car came from behind going sixty miles per hour rear-ended them.

Every sign triggered another call.

Over the course of the weekend, I drove on that same freeway three times roundtrip, each time the volume and intensity of my memories turned up a notch. Being on the ice and playing hockey washed my mind of the haunting images, but only temporarily since I had to drive home.

With each sign I passed, the video came into sharper focus. By Sunday night on my drive home, my brain vibrated and I no longer saw the scenes from a distance. I no longer saw myself kneeling down to the mangled kid with a spotlight on him. I no longer pictured myself on the Carquinez Bridge trying to roll over a young man whose pelvis felt like it had broken into hundreds of pieces.

I didn't "see," but in my head I walked on that bridge. I stood outside that children's hospital and heard the mom scream. I knelt in the gravel by the side of the road, trying to decide who to intubate first.

Only fifteen minutes from home, I hit my breaking point. I started to hyperventilate and sweat. My heart pounded and my teeth clenched and . . .

Shut it off! Shut it off!

My eyes scanned the road for a tree. A big tree. A big tree where I could build up a lot of speed and turn this off.

Everything in my head moved faster and louder and brighter and . . . *Igottafindatreeenowstopthisnowholdonchristyholdonchristyareonly10minutesfromhome.*

Fuuuuccckkkk!

My face was pouring sweat now. I drove faster.

Theeucalyptusinthemiddleofthehilljustholdonjustholdon. TheresaguywhosebodyfaceandheadisamangledmessandthereisaspotlightonhimFuck.

Okayokayokayonly5minutesfromhomealmosthomealmosthomejustkeepgoing.

I pulled into my driveway so fast that I almost drove through the garage door. I opened my car door, slid out, and bent over, my hands on my knees, trying to breathe.

When I gathered myself enough to put the key in the lock and walk through the front door, the house was dark except for the one light Lisa had left on for me. She was in bed, asleep already.

I collapsed on to the living room floor on my back. There I lay, exhausted, on the carpet like a pack of rabid wolves had chased me through an open field, and I'd just barely escaped. The wolves had been this close to ripping me apart, and no one had heard my screams.

CHAPTER TWENTY-NINE

It was the end of January and my QME appointment loomed. As each moment passed, the weight of the appointment became heavier. I felt like my life depended on the outcome of this meeting. A single person held my future in her hands. She was to determine for workers' comp whether I really had PTSD, and if so, if I'd gotten it from the job.

The day before my QME appointment, I ran errands to keep my mind busy. Just as I walked out of a coffee shop, my phone rang. Dr. Turner, the psychologist who would be doing my QME, called. She asked if it was okay if she brought her therapy dog, Harvey, to the meeting.

"I find many of my clients really enjoy having Harvey there," she said. "You don't have a problem with dogs, do you?"

I do like dogs, but it was such a leading question, I knew better than to say "no." I wasn't sure I wanted her dog there, but this lady held my entire future in her hands. Her findings and report would be a final decision.

"Sure. I like dogs," I said.

"And you might want to bring a sandwich," she said. "These things tend to take several hours."

The QME letter stated I would be charged if I didn't show up on time. I pulled up to a three-story wooden office building tucked in the back of a shopping center. I arrived early, so I sat in my car, becoming more and more nervous. Finally, it was time. My sweaty armpits and I opened the glass front door, went inside, and knocked on her office door.

No one answered. I walked back to the waiting area and sat down in a yellow vinyl chair. And waited. My leg jack hammered, my palms were sweaty, and I fidgeted in the chair.

About fifteen minutes later, a middle-aged woman in black pants and a purple sweater, both decorated with dog hair, walked down the hallway with a happy, medium-sized Sheltie dog.

The woman had black-and-gray hair, which stuck out and up randomly, and a very sincere, warm smile. "Are you Christine Warren?" she asked.

"Yes, I am. Are you Dr. Turner?"

"I am. Welcome. If you give me a second, I will get myself organized and then you can come back."

A few minutes later, she brought me back to her office, which, like her clothes, was adorned with dog hair. I tried not to let my distaste show. I loved dogs, but I have never been a fan of having animal fur all over my clothes.

Dr. Turner chatted as she set up an old, small, rickety, wooden, TV-dinner stand. Out of her briefcase she pulled a twelve-inch, old, white MacBook. It took up almost the entire stand. She pressed the power button and her face lit up when the computer came on, as if this was a surprise. She kept chatting and dug through her briefcase. "Oh dear. Oh dear. I seem to have left the power cord at home." She continued to look for it and finally said, "Well, let's just hope I have enough battery left to finish."

We sat there as the old computer loaded. Each time the computer completed a step closer to getting to her template, Dr. Turner smiled a huge warm smile and apologized for the computer taking so long to load.

When she finally got started, she asked me several questions about me, my childhood, my family, my wife, my job, my PTSD, my symptoms, and how I spent my days.

About an hour into it, she said, "Hold on a second. Let me save what we have so far. I forgot to save an interview only once!"

Three hours later, the interview portion was over. Miraculously, Dr. Turner's computer had enough "juice" to last the whole interview.

She handed me a stack of papers consisting of personality tests—the Myers-Briggs, Minnesota Multiple Personality Inventory, a handful of smaller ones, and a pencil. "I have a client coming in, so I need you to go to the waiting room to do these tests."

"Ok . . . um . . . Can I have a clipboard or something to use to take these tests on?" Filling in bubbles would be tough to do on my knee.

"Oh, that's a good idea." She searched and found one. I headed out to the waiting room and sat down in the same yellow vinyl seat. I started the tests and shifted around in my chair to be moderately comfortable.

About an hour later, Dr. Turner came through the waiting room with Harvey on a leash that had a blue bag tied around it. "Well, I am taking Harvey out to do his business. He didn't do his business like he usually docs in the morning. He also needs to check his pee mail."

"Good luck," I said with lukewarm enthusiasm, while I continued to fill in small circles with a number 2 pencil.

When Dr. Turner returned, the blue bag was missing from Harvey's leash.

"Harvey checked all his pee mail and did his business!" she said cheerfully.

Her timing was impeccable; the next question on the test asked if I felt suicidal.

❧

Three weeks later, in mid-February, I found a large, thick manilla envelope crammed in my mailbox. Dr. Turner's return address showed in the upper left corner.

I carried the envelope that contained the decision of my future into my house. If it said I was full of crap, I would either have to go back to work or quit. If it said my PTSD was real and caused by my job, I would have time and continued resources to heal.

It was late afternoon and the sun had already passed by the windows in the dining room. I turned the overhead light on and sat at our large wooden dining room table and took a deep breath. I stuck my finger under and slid it along the envelope flap.

Like I was trying to solve a wordfinder puzzle, my eyes desperately searched the first page full of text for that one sentence. Right on the front page I found it.

"I conclude that the predominant cause of Ms. Warren's PTSD derives from the cumulative trauma as a firefighter and paramedic. Her case of PTSD represents a secondary or vicarious condition of a first responder dealing with horrific human experiences that occurred over a period of years."

With that one sentence, the fear of what would happen to me if I had to go back to work, drained out of my chest. Not moving from my chair, I read the words over and over. Now, I had a fighting chance . . . and validation, too.

Oh my God, I am not crazy. Up to the point of getting the report, I'd felt like a hired hit man had been following me, waiting for the opportunity to shoot me in the back as I tried to run from him. With this letter, it was like that person had disappeared in a puff of smoke. This was certified proof that what I'd experienced on the job had caused my distress.

For the first time since the PTSD diagnosis, I was able to breathe deeply.

A few hours later, when Lisa came home from work, I handed her the report. I was crying, but this time, I didn't ask why I was crying. This time the reason was abundantly clear. For the time being, I did not have to ready myself for work by putting my armor back on or building the wall back up.

But it wasn't all good feelings. I'd been standing with one foot still in the Berkeley Fire Department. As much as I feared for my life if I had to go back to work, I also wanted to go back to work. Now, with this QME finding, my foot had been cut from BFD, taking with it my security and identity.

If I'm not a firefighter anymore, who am I?

I had been so vigilant and on my guard to keep it all together in case I had to go back to my job, I began to release my hypervigilance. With letting it go, I realized how exhausted I was.

I felt certain sleep would come that night—but it didn't. I slept horribly, and brutal nightmares plagued me. I woke up at 2:30 a.m. and couldn't go back to sleep until around 5:00 a.m. When I got up, I was grumpy and shut down.

I was so tired of having a good day, only to fall flat on my face the next. I was tired of being weak, of not being able to go to work and do my job. I was tired of needing someone else to take care of me. My inner critic went on a rampage. *You are worthless, weak, and suck at everything,* it berated me.

After stewing all morning on how worthless I was, I went outside and washed my car. Anxiety and anger welled up inside of me. I threw the sponge and kicked the water bucket across the driveway.

Lisa stood in in the garage, watching me.

I said, "What in the fuck is wrong with me? Yesterday I felt good and today I am so defeated and angry!"

"Good days are usually followed by crappy ones," she said to me. "A bad day doesn't mean things are getting worse. In fact, you are having more good days."

Lisa didn't get mad or upset or try to further engage me on whether I was doing a good or bad job. She just stated the facts.

I don't know if her matter-of-fact ways would be helpful to everyone, but for me they made all the difference. She made it clear she knew my issues had nothing to do with her. There was nothing she did or didn't do that caused my anger or depression. Defused but exhausted, I spent the entire day at home, not talking. But Lisa's words helped me hold onto a small glimmer of hope that this was just one bad day.

It's not forever, I told myself. *More good days are to come.*

In the following days and weeks, I had more shitty days than good days. On one of those shitty days, I sat in my recliner at home, ruminating over the tennis match I'd just lost.

I couldn't even do tennis right. It was so important for me to win, to continue my desperate search for proof that I was a good person. My mind snapped to the loaded gun, locked in a safe in my closet. All I needed was my fingerprint to open the safe.

Just do it. I will just go into the garage and do it. This world will be so much better off without me.

I was so stuck in my thoughts, I couldn't get up out of my chair to get my gun. So I visualized putting the gun in my mouth and ending everything—my still body and silent head on the floor, my blood all over the wall. I'd be gone. Everything would be quiet. The worthless burden who'd failed would no longer cause misery to others. Everyone could take a deep breath and get back to their lives.

Finally, I got up out of the recliner and walked down the hall to my office. I slid open the closet door and rested my pointer finger on the gun safe fingerprint button. The lid softly and quietly opened, revealing a 9mm Glock. I picked it up and felt the weight in my hands. I no longer heard anything except the constant ringing in my ears.

I started down the hallway toward the garage. As I passed through the house, I saw everything Lisa had done for us. I loved our house. She had made such a comfortable, pleasant home for us.

I shouldn't do this. Tears ran down my face. I stopped with one hand on the doorknob to the garage and the other hand holding my gun. *I can't do this. I must get my shit together. I need help right now.*

I walked back into my office, anger surging in my head. I had failed another try to turn this shit off. I had to continue to live in this nightmare. I threw my gun across the room. Part of me hoped a round would go off and do what I couldn't find the courage to do. Tears poured down my face. *When is this going to stop?*

I returned to the living room and climbed back into the safety of my chair, then dialed Luke's, from WCPR, phone number.

"How goes it, Christy?"

"Not so good," I said. "Can I ask you a question?"

"Of course."

"When do you stop wanting to kill yourself?"

"Ah . . . it took me a long time. I felt like I didn't want to be here anymore all the time. Every time I made a mistake. Every time my wife got mad at me. For me, it stopped when I found Jesus Christ. I know that's not for everyone, but for me, that was it. I started finding other ways to deal with my feelings and eventually changed my thought process. You will get through it and the feelings will go away if you keep working at this. PTSD is hard. I had a good friend who had PTSD and then had cancer.

He said he would choose cancer over PTSD any day. But I promise, these feelings will stop."

When I told Luke later how thankful I was that he answered the phone—and let him know how close I was when I called him—he said I hadn't needed to tell him. He'd known; he could hear it in my voice. Luckily, after working with so many other first responders with PTSD, he knew exactly what to say to help me.

Once in bed, I wrote in my journal about needing to draw a line in the sand that I would no longer consciously choose to step over. All of this back and forth of being okay and then suddenly going dark wasn't serving me well. I had to stop the cycle. My heart wanted to get better, but my head did not believe I deserved to. I had to decide and make a choice to give myself a break. Feeling better about myself wasn't going to just happen. People had been telling me for years I was a good person, which obviously hadn't worked. I had to consciously keep telling myself I was a good person.

Barb used to say, "Change your self-talk and change your life."

After sorting this all out in my journal, I picked up the phone, which now felt like four hundred pounds instead of five hundred and called Barb.

"Hey Barb. I am so sorry to bother you. But you should be proud of me for actually calling you."

She said, "I am. What's going on?"

"I'm drowning. I can't stop thinking about suicide. I feel like I'm right back where I started . . . frustrated, hopeless, angry, and alone. There's nothing but chaos in my head."

She said, "Why don't we meet at the retreat and we can talk in person? Maybe being up there will help you remember how good you felt during the retreat."

We picked a time to meet the next day.

When I got there late morning, I was the only one on the property. I drank in the stillness and safety of the site—magic mountain as many WCPR alums call it.

About twenty minutes later, Barb pulled into the parking area. She got out of her truck and walked toward me. She gave me a big hug, and we sat down in front of the retreat building.

"Tell me, what's been going on."

Tears came the moment she asked the question. "I feel so hopeless. I am racked with anxiety and feeling shitty again. I was feeling so much better, and now it's all gone to shit. I'm failing!"

Barb replied, "You can do this. You are right where you are supposed to be. I know you can do this because I was able to. When I came through the retreat, I was an absolute mess."

Barb then shared with me the details of her own PTSD story, which I had never heard. By sharing her full story, I had proof, which for me equaled hope, that this shit could be overcome.

We talked for two hours. Once again, the magic place on the mountain reminded me I was not alone. When we finished, I felt like I'd gotten a booster shot of love and hope, which was exactly what I needed. PTSD had a way of stomping out any hope I could have, leaving me with no way through. With Barb's help, I'd revived my hope, and I could once again believe my miserable PTSD symptoms would not last forever.

I drove directly to San Rafael from the retreat center for a meeting with Linda Brown, now my official attorney. About a week prior, I had received a letter stating I would have to be deposed by a lawyer from ACS. Linda wanted to go over what I should expect at the deposition.

"You'll be deposed by the attorney representing workers' comp," Linda said, once we were in her office.

"Why do they need to depose me?"

"They're defending themselves to get out of the claim."

This seemed outrageous to me, given my QME report. How could they argue with the facts?

The anticipation of talking about this stuff in a threatening environment caused me great anxiety. ACS had required me to sign off to send their investigators my psychiatric notes, medical records, QME notes, my therapist's notes, and my credit report. They knew the details of every blood test, X-ray, doctor's visit, and gynecological exam. They read every detail of my visits with my therapist, where I once thought were sacred words between only me and Grace. They were allowed access to every detail of my life. They could use the fact I was molested as a child against me.

I battled this anxiety as Linda and I talked about the rules and what to expect during the deposition. Linda knew the opposing lawyer and shared with me he was a good person. "He'll do his job but won't be trying to make a fool outta you or tear you down. You sure lucked out getting him."

While good, this did little to lower my apprehension. This guy could make everything so much worse.

I tried to keep myself busy for the next week. But at night, in bed, I couldn't stop the nightmares. Each one began with me at work. In one, I received a phone call telling me to pick up my nieces and take them home. I got into my car, still in my uniform, and picked them up. Suddenly we were on a dirt road in the middle of a desert. We hit a rut in the road, and our car veered off the side and into a lake. Cold water rushed into the car like a broken dam. I screamed at the girls to take off their seatbelts, but the water poured in too fast. We were underwater. I swam into the back seat desperately trying to get the girls out while the car sank. My throat spasmed, and I knew if I didn't come up for air, I would drown, and I wouldn't be able to save them. I frantically swam to the surface for air before diving back to the car. No matter what I did, I couldn't get the girls out. The car continued to sink in the bottomless lake and when I swam back up to the surface, I screamed.

Lisa tried to hold me and stop me from thrashing. "It's okay. It's okay!"

I was wet, breathing like I really had been underwater, holding my breath. In every nightmare, I was responsible for rescuing someone.

I always failed.

CHAPTER THIRTY

In the beginning of March, I needed to experience something new and different—something to break the monotony of being home, going to therapy and lawyer appointments, the same routine, every day and every week.

Tom, one of my friends from the retreat, lived in Arizona and so did the Grand Canyon, which I'd never been to. I'd only seen pictures of it. The drive across the desert alone would be exhilarating.

Around 7:45 a.m. on March 9, 2015, I kissed Lisa goodbye, hopped in my Acura, and started my drive to Arizona.

As soon as I hit the onramp, I started crying. For twenty minutes, I could barely see through the salty water pooling in my eyes, a mixture of heartbreak and thrills.

When I finally made it to the Holiday Inn in Williams, Arizona, at 9:00 p.m., I was exhausted from the twelve-hour drive. Once in the quiet hotel room, PTSD noise bounced around in my head. I was all by myself. Still scared. Still anxious. Still uncertain of my future. But my goal on this trip was to be with myself and learn to accept the real me, whoever that was.

With my nightly cocktail of meds, sleep came swiftly, but the nightmares followed me to Arizona. All night I couldn't stop a couple of BFD firefighters from being blown up, despite my efforts. I woke up screaming and soaking wet with failure wrapped around me.

The next morning, the Grand Canyon pulled at me like an industrial strength magnet to get up and out of bed. I shoved some hotel-lobby extra-hard-boiled eggs into my mouth, poured myself some crappy coffee to go, and headed out the door.

Dirt and scrub trees surrounded the road on the way to the Grand Canyon. My anticipation crescendoed—and then crashed. All the signs said I had arrived. But first I had to circle the giant parking lot and find a parking space like it was a week before Christmas at the mall.

People milled everywhere. I guessed I would share my individual, spiritual experience with a few thousand other tourists. Once parked, I almost ran to the edge of the canyon. I stood and looked down at the expansive hole in the earth, matching the tip of my toes with the very edge. I could feel the earth breathe.

I could also smell the bathroom from where I stood, so I moved.

I walked along the asphalt path where I took advantage of every opportunity I found to step right up to the edge. Every time I peered over the canyon, I was in speechless awe. I experienced a connection to the earth I'd never felt before. The chasm before me looked like one of those boring-on-the-outside quartz rocks, which was beautiful on the inside. Something stirred in my soul.

I found a trailhead and walked down to the insides of the earth. What amazing beauty I found at the Grand Canyon. The silence stunned me. The air held an energy I could feel. When I found a quiet spot to sit, a crow flew over my head. With each flap of its wings, I heard the air rip apart.

Feeling energized, I stood up, dusted myself off, and continued down the staircase of earth. The farther I walked, the more relief I felt. Quiet. My head was quiet. The air was quiet. The quiet wrapped around me like a blanket, keeping me safe and warm. I focused on sounds around me instead of sounds inside my head. The magnitude of the canyon gave me the sense of being a part of something bigger than myself and no longer alone. A giddy happiness replaced my anxiety—from being there and getting myself there. I felt good, hopeful, content, worthy, and present. I was tired, but it was a good kind of tired.

I found the perfect spot to witness the sunset. I hiked to get away from all the people and found a spot on the edge. The setting sun and the canyon assembled in perfect juxtaposition. From this vantage point, I witnessed the earth rotating away from the sun.

I waited until the Earth had spun completely away and the sky turned a dark, royal blue dotted with stars. Then I rose, walked back to the now empty parking lot, and climbed into my car.

As I drove back to my hotel on the two-lane highway, the darkness intensified the proximity of vehicles speeding by each other. After ten minutes, car wrecks from the last twenty-five years poured in.

My whole body flinched. Feelings of peace and visions of holy ground suddenly switched to wrecked cars, bloodied and mangled people, and furious noise. My hope and stillness became misery and chaos.

I talked myself through the rest of the drive. "My name is Christy Warren and I have PTSD. I need to behave my way through this. That means cry when I feel the need to cry." This self-talk sustained me all the way back to the hotel. It was like living each sentence at a time. And I wasn't sure if the tears would ever turn off.

That night I wrote in my journal, "This will not last forever!"

The next morning, it took a minute to figure out where I was. The tears started back up and would not stop. Visions of wrecks and people I frantically tried to save but could not overwhelmed me.

A whisper blew through my head. *Do something.*

I picked up my phone and called Barb. She talked me out of the glue I stood in and got me to move.

"Behave your way out. Take action," she said. She then suggested I write what was in my heart.

As soon as we hung up, I started writing:

March 10, 2015

To everyone I couldn't save:

I am so sorry. I am so sorry. I am so sorry. I cry rivers of tears for you. I dream about you. I replay your tragedy over and over in my mind. It makes my heart ache. There are so many of you, but each one of you is so unique. I remember your faces, your mangled parts, and your devastated families, and I am so sorry. It was my job to fix you enough for you to be sent back home to your life, your husbands, your wives, and your partners. What are your children going to do without you? I am so sorry. If I could fix all of you, I would. But I can't.

I hope you knew I was there for you, even in your horrible death. I hope you were able to feel my presence, my genuine care and compassion for you. Oh my God there were so many of you.

I am human. I have made mistakes. I cannot apologize enough. But I promise you I gave you my best I had at the time. You all deserve the best.

To the woman whose baby I couldn't save. I am so sorry. The pain within your scream remains with me. I will never forget.

To the man on Oregon St., who I was supposed to find but didn't, because I got sidetracked by a shiny object, I will forever be sorry.

—Christy

After writing the letter, I could finally breathe. I couldn't believe the power of putting the words on the page.

Just then, my phone dinged.

Tom had sent a text to our entire retreat group. "What happened to Christy, did she jump?"

I laughed my ass off. I wrote back, "I am too pathetic right now to jump because I can't even get off the floor. I am crying my eyes out in the corner of my room." I don't know exactly why Tom made me laugh so hard, but between him and writing the letter, a tremendous weight fell off me and blew to dust when it hit the ground. Elated to spend another day at the Grand Canyon, and to see Tom that night, I packed up, threw on some clothes, and headed out the door.

Tom lived in a tiny town in the middle of a forest. Our first day together, we went to a San Francisco Giants spring training game, something I had always wanted to do.

On the way to the stadium, we drove through the city where Tom used to be a cop. He pointed out every street corner, building, sidewalk, and intersection where he had encountered a horrific call. Tom's face tightened up, and his eyes focused when he said, "Here is where I pulled a woman out of a burning car, but I couldn't get the rest of her family out."

I felt his anguish, but by the time we got to the game, a smile was back on his face and his eyes had lightened up.

During my visit, we spent some time with the love of Tom's life, his eight-year-old grandson. Tom would play and banter with him as if he was a kid himself.

I watched Tom with his grandson. Tom had an amazing, loving, and tender heart. He had such an incredible capacity to love and be good to whatever and whomever needed it. But when your life is threatened, he was the guy you wanted coming to the house to kick down the front door and save everyone. We had that in common. *No wonder we both got PTSD,* I thought. A tender, loving heart can only withstand so much tragedy and so much pain while shoving every "normal" reaction away.

Recognizing that strength and being good at the job can cause PTSD, I began to understand I was not weak nor did having PTSD mean I was a bad person.

What a trip.

What a fantastic, hard, lonely, full-of-discovery, heart-filling, grieving, fast, long, and amazing trip. I couldn't wait to get home to see my wife—my wonderful, loving, flawed, smart, introverted, patient, amazing wife whose smile lit up the room . . . and my heart.

CHAPTER THIRTY-ONE

I couldn't wait for March 22, the Sunday afternoon I got to go back to WCPR as a peer. But once I arrived and walked through the door, I wanted to get back in my car and drive home. My body fought against the gaping hole of vulnerability this place created, and I knew I needed to talk about that fire, about how I'd fucked up that day.

What if I tell everyone who I really am? How I have no business being a captain? What if all this love and acceptance I have found gets ripped out from under me when they know?

I was terrified. But if I was ever going to get out from under this heavy blanket of shame, I had to come clean.

Once the clients marched to the Rubber Room to vomit their shitty traumas and misery all over each other, the peers sat in a circle in the living room to talk. It was now Tuesday, our first peer gathering. One peer talked about struggling with his anxiety and nightmares. Another talked about his wife leaving him because she just couldn't take it anymore. He said he didn't blame her, since he'd been a nightmare to live with. Then it was my turn.

My eyes welled up. *For fuck's sake, Christy, can't you not cry just once?* I gathered myself and told the entire story—every honest piece of my mistake at the Oregon Street fire. Everyone in the room listened intently, and no one thought I failed. Everyone said what I already knew—the guy was dead already. Two engine companies plus the truck did not find him, either.

I'd hope that finally sharing this story would relieve the weight of my guilt. But even with all the positive feedback I was given, I kept trying to confirm the negative. I assured myself that they just said what they felt obliged to say, not what they believed—I sucked as a firefighter and even more as a captain. They were just doing what so many of us first responders do—fixing the problem. The ball of shame still kneeled on my chest.

Jay Scott spoke. He was a retired Oklahoma City firefighter, who was one of the first people on the scene of the Oklahoma City bombing. I had a deep respect for him, since he was genuine, kind, and held high standards.

He leaned in toward me and said, "You know how I know you aren't a failure? Because I also did the unthinkable, and I'm not a failure."

He sat up straight, and his voice relayed confidence and compassion. He did not speak with anger or self-hate. Jay told his story of committing the "unthinkable" during the bombing. He and his crew were in the middle of the rubble and those in charge of the incident suddenly believed they'd found a secondary device and set off the alarms for everyone to abandon the area. He felt a great pull to stay, and he told us what he thought.

"So many victims remained inside. What if they see everyone who came to rescue them suddenly run away? It went against every fiber of my being."

But the higher-ups insisted he leave. Finally, and begrudgingly, he ran. The gravity of the situation caught up with him, and he ran for his life. While running, he had to jump from a sizeable chunk of concrete. As he leapt from the debris, his eye caught a woman crumpled on the ground just below the concrete. As he jumped over her, he saw she was pregnant. Still, his adrenaline and orders from higher rank kept him running. To him, she appeared to be dead, but he didn't know for sure.

Jay looked right into my eyes and said, "This moment haunted me for years. I had to learn to forgive and have compassion for myself. It took a while but shit, I am only human. You need to realize that, too."

If Jay, a brave and strong firefighter, could forgive himself for what he'd done, maybe I could, too. Maybe I owed myself the same grace and compassion.

During the retreat, I made another ever-so-slight shift. While eating snacks in the living room with several peers, one of them made a positive comment about me. I immediately shut him down. The critical asshole who rented out an apartment in my head spoke out loud and would not let me hear the kind comment.

When I did that, Lou squinted at me and said, "You can choose to listen to the voices who tell you that you are a piece of shit, or you can listen to those who love you and care about you or even those who barely even know you and think you are a good person."

Everyone looked at me, and a few voices spoke up to agree with Lou. I was shamed into being good to myself. I promised to choose to listen to those who loved and cared about me instead of the asshole in my head.

It was at least a start.

On the last evening of the retreat, a psychiatrist spoke to us about medication for PTSD—something that usually happened at the retreats but hadn't taken place at mine.

First responders, for the most part, view taking psych medications as a weakness, like it's a crutch. We believe we must be strong and can get through the madness without medications. It's like refusing pain meds for an injury. We're not so different from little kids whose parents offer to help them do something, and they say, "No! I can do this myself."

The doctor, who wore a T-shirt that said, "Unfuck the world," spoke with a matter-of-fact voice as if the information she was presenting should be well known. But it wasn't because the system had failed to educate us.

"Taking medication for PTSD is no different from taking insulin for diabetes," she said. "PTSD is a biological injury to your brain. A brain scan will look different between people who have PTSD and those who don't."

She continued to talk about the different PTSD medications. She had some of us act out the effects of a broken pancreas, which could not produce insulin.

Three volunteers stood in a circle holding hands, representing a cell wall. One person stood inside the circle—a single cell. One person stood outside the circle—a molecule of glucose. The last person—insulin—stood several feet back from the cell wall.

In the first scenario, the glucose molecule tried to get through the cell wall and into the cell. The cell wall held their hands tightly together and would not let the glucose cell in. A superhero insulin approached the cell wall and exclaimed, "Do not fret glucose! I will get you through the cell wall and into the cell."

The doctor had insulin break apart one set of holding hands to allow glucose to enter the cell. Then, looking perplexed, she asked the room, "Now why would someone whose pancreas doesn't produce insulin not take insulin? Would it be because they worried about what people thought? Or because taking insulin is weak and you don't want to be a pussy?"

No one said a thing.

She surveyed the room. "PTSD is the same thing! You have a

chemical imbalance in your brain, just like the body has a chemical imbalance in someone who has diabetes. Taking medication isn't a crutch or being weak. Your brain needs these chemicals to function properly."

There was no sales pitch, just the facts and the attitude she projected. Peers and clients asked the doctor a lot of specific questions. Almost all the peers were on PTSD medications—Zoloft, Paxil, Effexor, Wellbutrin, and other meds to treat the symptoms of PTSD and depression.

Instead of feeling like the tough person who belonged with this group, I felt like the idiot the psychologist was talking about.

After the talk, a few of us discussed taking meds. I asked one of my tough-as-nails, working-cop peers, "*You* are taking meds? Really?"

He replied, "I sure am. They really help, and I can still work while on them."

A seed of possibility was planted in my brain. Maybe taking meds would be okay. Taking them didn't mean I was weak or a failure.

When I got home Friday afternoon, feeling exhausted but relieved, I found another letter from workers' comp awaiting me.

March 25, 2015

Dear Ms. Warren:

After receipt of all available information, we have accepted your claim in regard to the above injury.

Please be informed that we will provide benefits for all authorized medical treatment and prescribed medications. We also will reimburse you for all mileage traveled to and from treating doctors and physical therapy treatments, upon submission of your request for reimbursement.

For your protection, California law requires the following to appear on this form: "Any person who knowingly present a false or fraudulent claim for the payment of a loss is guilty of a crime and may be subject to fines and confinement in state prison."

Well, thank you ACS. The irony wasn't lost on me. Now that I was doing better, they'd finally accepted my claim. Again, the thought occurred to me they were hoping I would kill myself before they had to accept my claim. I was in awe of the lengths they'd go to in order to not have to pay for my treatment.

I also found it ironic that they delivered the good news while threatening fines and prison.

The very next day, I received a letter from Linda Brown. I stood in the street in front of the row of green mailboxes and opened the letter. The first page was official-looking. In big letters it read, "City of Berkeley Fire Department V. Christine Warren."

I knew it was just a legal formality, but reading the words felt like a punch in the teeth. I was just trying to keep myself alive and my department was taking me to court to dispute my claim that I had gotten PTSD on the job. Also in the envelope was my attorney/client agreement, which stated, "This firm will request an attorney fee of 15% to 18% of the benefits awarded or obtained."

What a waste! The combined amount of money workers' comp was blowing and what I would lose was ridiculous! I was entering into this ordeal with such negative feelings just when I was trying to commit myself to getting better.

CHAPTER THIRTY-TWO

On April 6, the day of my deposition, Lisa drove me to Linda's office in San Rafael. We arrived early for some deposition prep.

My prep included Linda Brown reminding me again, "Do not lie!" Her face came very close to mine, as did her pointer finger. She repeated, "Do not ever lie. And don't give them any more information than asked for. Answer exactly what they are asking in their question. If they want more information, they will ask." She pointed at me. "By the way, we called Berkeley Fire to see what's in your file and what they thought of you. Did you know they think very highly of you? They said you are honest and hold yourself accountable."

"They did?" A solid, smooth piece of validation settled into the bottom of my chest, in the very moment I needed it most.

From Linda's office, Lisa and I walked down to the conference room together. My insides danced and tangled among each other. A Tasmanian devil fighting to the death used my stomach for an arena. I couldn't sit down.

On the first floor of the office building, the dark conference room took up the far end of the open-floor plan. A pieced-together glass wall separated the conference room and the rest of the large downstairs room. The little kid in me was pretty sure the boogeyman man lurked inside. I refused to go in there until I had to.

About fifteen minutes later, Linda came down and the three of us waited for the opposing attorney to arrive.

Breaking the silence, Linda asked, "So, what kind of tennis do you play?"

"Mostly singles, but I play doubles, too."

"Do you play 'sorry' tennis?"

"What's that?"

"That's the kind of tennis I play . . . because I'm always saying 'sorry' for screwing up all the time."

I chuckled as she described my tennis abilities perfectly. "Oh yeah, I play a lot of 'sorry' tennis."

Linda was the type of person to ask random questions, which lowered the temperature in the room. She made me laugh despite the seriousness of the situation and the anxiety wrapped around me like a serpent crushing my lungs.

We kept waiting. The silence grew thick again, clouded with Linda's impatience and my anxiety. Linda called her daughter and had her usual spirited short-and-to-the-point conversation with her. Then Linda called upstairs, short and to the point. "Where in the hell is Ken Christopher?!"

After a few phone calls back and forth, we found out the deposition had been canceled. It would be rescheduled for a later date.

Linda was furious. I was relieved.

CHAPTER THIRTY-THREE

From almost the beginning of therapy, Grace would ask, "Have you thought any more about meds?"

Each time I responded, "You know the answer to that. I'm not taking meds."

Now, a year after being diagnosed with PTSD and a few months after the psychiatrist gave the talk about PTSD medications at the retreat, I sat at my dining room table, paralyzed by my anxiety and the noise and scenes playing in my head. My head rested on my hands like a pillow on the table.

I feel like I've been kicked to the bottom of a hole. The lights have been shut off. Monsters lurk, and the walls are electrified. I can't get any lower than this. I cannot feel any worse than this. I might as well try meds. I have nothing to lose because I am sure I cannot feel any shittier than I do now.

Just then, Lisa walked into the room. I lifted my head off the table and said, "Well, fuck this. I can't tell you how horrible I feel right now. I might as well try meds."

"I think that's an excellent idea," she said.

She had been advocating that I go on meds since all of this started.

I ignored the sarcasm, grabbed my phone, and called Grace.

"Grace. I can't take this anymore. I have nothing to lose, so I am ready to try meds."

She quickly replied, "Oh Christy I'm so sorry you feel like this, but I am very happy, and rather surprised that you are finally going to try medication. I will call Dr. Jankovic right away."

A few minutes later she called me back and told me I had an appointment with Dr. Jankovic the next day.

I walked into the waiting room to sit in my usual waiting-room chair, the farthest in the back against the wall, facing the door. Grace and Dr. Jankovic's offices shared a waiting room. Dr. Jankovic, tall, blond, and easy on the eyes had a joyful smile on a serious face. She spoke with an Eastern European accent. She gave me 100 percent of her attention and listened with the intensity of a surgeon performing brain surgery.

It was clear to me she deeply cared about her patients. She asked tough questions and asked about the smallest details, including the times I'd felt suicidal. We talked about my drinking with no judgment from her. She was fiercely protective, and I knew she would not let me slip out of her sight.

At the beginning of the session, I'd signed all the release forms, so she'd connected with Grace before my appointment. I'd given them permission to consult with one another about my treatment.

She brought up my guns and said, "You have to put your guns in the care of someone else. After you get home, I want Lisa to call me to confirm you gave them up."

I stayed quiet for a minute as my thoughts cycled from *That's ridiculous!* to *How embarrassing!* to *Yeah, she's right.*

We talked about different medications for PTSD. She highly suggested Seroquel, but one of its potential side effects was diabetes.

I said, "No thank you. I don't need PTSD and diabetes."

We discussed a ton of medication options and ultimately decided on Paxil. Paxil sounded like it would give me the greatest relief with the least amount of side effects.

I had heard many other first responders with PTSD say how they'd have an appointment, get a prescription, and be on their way with no follow up appointment or even a phone call. But Dr. Jankovic wanted me back the next week. I saw her every week for a month and then every other week for several months. She never let me down.

On May 5, 2015, after I'd been on Paxil for just over two weeks, my rescheduled deposition day arrived. Once again, Lisa drove us to Linda Brown's office in San Rafael. Lisa and I walked to the conference room in my attorney's building. My insides twisted into a compressed mess. I picked a chair with my back to the wall facing the door. Lisa waited for me on a couch outside the conference room, where a gas fireplace burned on the lower half and a large, flat screen TV displayed a tropical fish tank on top. Linda Brown jokingly called it the Fish Fry room.

One-inch spacers separated each sheet of glass between the Fish Fry room and the conference room. Everything could be overheard in the conference room. During the deposition, I knew Lisa intently listened to every word spoken.

Linda and the court reporter arrived at the same time. The enormous conference room was big enough for twenty-five people. As Linda sat down next to me on the right, she chucked a yellow pad of paper onto the table. The court reporter sat to my left, at the head of the table. The opposing attorney arrived next, wearing a salmon-colored polo shirt.

This was the guy Linda had told me was a good person. I hoped it held true today.

He came in relaxed and smiling, like he'd done this a thousand times before. He introduced himself as Ken. He and Linda shared friendly sarcastic banter while he organized his paperwork.

Even though I felt his easiness and kindness, it didn't stop me from crying before we got started. I put my head down on the table to gather my shit together. I didn't know what was coming next. The devil fought inside me and I thought I would vomit. *I don't want to talk about what a failure I am. I don't want to talk with some stranger about being molested, especially when it has nothing to do with my PTSD. We all know I am defective, and I can't handle my job, so do we really need to keep talking about it?*

Linda patted me on the back and said, "My God, you are going to be fine. Trust me."

I took a deep breath and wiped the snot and tears from my face onto my sleeve.

Ken gave me my instructions. I was not to answer his question until he completely finished asking it. I failed at this miserably. I answered his questions like I was a contestant on a game show. I just wanted it over. He had to constantly remind me to wait.

He led me through a series of questions from broad to specific, which included my injuries. When we got to my knees, I told him how my orthopedic doctor told me I have "firefighter's knees" from carrying heavy loads up and down stairs.

Linda was excited. "Did you hear that, Ken? Those were the doctor's exact words. 'firefighter's knees.'" She wrote "firefighter's knees" on her yellow legal pad.

"Yeah, I heard it," Ken said. He asked me to clear up a few things from my therapist's notes and then informed me the insurance company would accept my claim.

"And will you just pay these damn bills?" Linda said.

"Yes," he said, "we will pay her bills."

A wave of relief and exhaustion fell over me. I had heard so many horror stories, I had prepared for the firing squad to put a hood over my head and yell, "Fire!"

∽

A week after letting go of so much angst, a routine trip to the mailbox piled the angst back on.

Dear Ms. Warren,

Although liability for your workers' compensation injury has been accepted, I cannot pay your benefits at this time because we need to coordinate the payment of this benefit with your employer and your long-term disability carrier. I expect to advise you of the status of these benefits by 5/24/15.

I shook my head in disbelief. If I was supporting a family, I would have likely lost my house or killed myself by now. How could the system be so broken?

CHAPTER THIRTY-FOUR

I aimlessly wandered through the rest of May. All my days were the same. I saw Grace, Caroline, and my psychiatrist. I ran. I stared at the walls and paced around the house. The meds decreased my anxiety, but they didn't stop the nightmares. I still struggled, believing my only worth was in being a firefighter. If I tried harder, I could outrun the pain.

To improve my symptoms, Dr. Jankovic increased my Paxil dose, but this made me drowsy, so I backed off the dosage to where it had been before. She tried prescribing Prazosin to stop the nightmares. I was hopeful the Prazosin would work, as it worked for so many people. But the first night I took it, the nightmares increased. She took me off the Prazosin and pre-scribed Topamax for the nightmares.

Like a miracle, the Topamax worked, and the nightmares stopped. I called it "Topamarbegone." But after taking it for a few weeks, I became forgetful and walked through the day with my brain in a fog.

One day Lisa said to me, "I hope you won't be driving with your nieces in the car while you are on this."

The next time I saw Dr. Jankovic, I brought this up, and we both agreed I should stop taking Topamax. It wasn't worth it.

❧

Lisa stood by me through all of it: the temper tantrums, the not being present, the having to watch me every minute of the day because she feared for my safety. She always made it clear she knew my craziness had nothing to do with her. I did not have to explain myself to her or take care of her. This allowed me to focus on getting better and was a tremendous relief, given all the other stresses in my life.

In early June 2015, eight months after I had left work, I called Drew, my close friend from work, who'd pranked me in the past by holding the chainsaw to my leg, and asked him if we could meet for coffee.

When we met, I said, "I just want to explain why I didn't reach out to you."

His expression indicated whatever I said wouldn't justify my absence.

"The shame consumed me. It paralyzed me. You are someone who I respect so much and only dream I could be half the firefighter you are. You are the toughest person I know, and I felt like a fraud."

"I thought we were better friends than that," he said.

"I didn't talk to anyone. I didn't even know what was going on with me. I was a mess."

"It sounds like you're asking for my forgiveness," he said.

"I am."

"You don't need my forgiveness. You do what you need to do. It is what it is."

I wasn't exactly sure what Drew meant. I was worried about saying the wrong thing. I valued our friendship tremendously, and I didn't know how else to repair it.

We stared into our coffees for a few minutes in silence. After sipping his coffee, Drew asked me some questions about the workers' comp process.

"Well I am glad to know there is a process in place in case this happens to me."

We finished our coffee and left. Drew never spoke to me again. I was hurt but understood. I was learning the hard way that PTSD leaves a path of destruction. It destroys marriages, ruins parents' relationships with their children, and ruins friendships. Some of it can be repaired and some cannot. The shame and fear of PTSD feels like life and death, as if someone stood on a tightrope and had to remain focused forward as to not let anything push them. The smallest push further into shame or fear could literally cause your death. Workers' comp was so detrimental. When help was finally requested, the system fed the shame.

The day finally came when Lisa couldn't keep it all stuffed inside anymore.

"I've never been so lonely in all my life," she said to me through tears. "For the past two years, everything has been about you. I can't even spend time with my friends because I can't take my eyes off you for a minute. I'm lonely. And I'm tired. I am so unhappy."

She had been patient with me, not taking my emotional absence personally, watching me all the time, putting up with my totally unpredictable anger and moodiness, knowing I was lying to her by drinking when she wasn't looking. Even so, I was stunned when she finally broke down.

I completely understood, but I also didn't know what to do.

"I will figure this out," I said. "Just please don't leave me."

The words *I'm so fucked* flooded my mind. I had no job. I couldn't get a job since it would completely forfeit my workers' comp claim. I could barely walk from my hip surgery. My brain was a mess. I had become something I swore I would never, ever become: a burden. I was causing the person I loved most in the world pain. How had I turned into this person?

Lisa stopped talking, and I just kept apologizing.

"I'll figure this out," I repeated like a broken record. "I'll fix it."

Lisa went outside to mow the lawn. Her mind and thoughts always turned inside while her body always went outside to process something and think.

I stared out the window, trying to push my tears back. I went to my desk and allowed my tears to overcome me. I reached for the box of Kleenex, which had been given to me from my friends at WCPR, and read their signatures. These guys were my saving grace. This was exactly why I'd brought the box home. For this moment, when desperation took hold. I had to keep going for these guys.

I called Tom. "Dude, I feel horrible. I don't want to be here anymore. I don't want this crap in my head anymore. I just want to end it."

Tom said, "You can't. It'll destroy the group. Each of us keeping our heads above keeps us all going. So, you just can't."

A quiet fell between us as I thought about what he had said.

"I get it. You are right. I know how I'd feel if someone else in our group did it. I know I can't do that to any of us. Thank you."

Between Tom's words and the Kleenex box, I had a small smile on my face by the time I hung up the phone. I finally wanted to come out of isolation.

Lisa was watching TV when I entered the living room. She had processed what she was feeling while outside, and I processed mine by talking to Tom. We sat quietly together on the couch. *Sixty Minutes* was on the TV. They were doing a story called "Life After Death Row," featuring Anthony Ray Hinton, who had spent thirty years on death row in a small cell, waiting for his turn in the electric chair. The story was about his exoneration, after the courts had revisited his case thirty years later.

Hinton survived those thirty isolated and lonely years by monitoring the dialogue in his head. He spoke of kindness, gratitude, and compassion. His story was one of gratitude instead of anger, of not wasting one more day stuck in the past.

Hinton's words hit me hard. *Changing the dialogue in my head could change my life.* I needed a new way to look at life. I had so much to be grateful for. I had work to do.

For a week I'd been mentally rehearsing picking up all my shit from Station 6.

I had been scared to get my stuff for a long time. As long as my gear still hung on the racks next to the engine in the apparatus bay, I belonged. But it was past time to go. I had been gone long enough that my position on the engine had opened up. I needed to get my gear out of the way for the new captain.

I knew I was never going back. Station 6 would be my last home at Berkeley Fire.

I'd picked a day when I knew Wyatt, a friend and coworker I trusted, would be on duty.

"Please come down for lunch," he'd said. "We will take care of it."

Lisa and several other friends offered to go with me, but I wanted to go alone. I wanted to savor those last moments of being a part of something I needed and loved before I erased myself from that world.

Grace often told me to picture everyone who loved me, holding me up when I felt scared and alone. Before I climbed into the car to make the last drive to Berkeley, I concentrated on the love and support from those who'd been holding me up.

When I arrived at Station 6, the engine was out. The gate

code to the parking area was the same, so I parked in the back of the station. But the station door code no longer worked. I was going to have to wait for the engine to return.

I stood in front of the door, defeated, like an outsider. *I used to belong here*, I thought. Then I found a positive thought and called one of my coworker pals for the code. He gave it to me, and I went inside the apparatus bay.

Thankful for the solitude, I closed my eyes and smelled the air of the apparatus floor. Oil, omex, structure fire smoke, and mildew. I savored the heaviness of my turnout coat. I grabbed my helmet by the front shield and put it on my head, leaving the chin strap loose, just like we wore them. I have a tiny head and I've always looked like I was a kid wearing my dad's hat when I put on my helmet, and I allowed a small smile at the image of myself.

My brain vacillated between false hopes of going back to work and knowing I would never go back. I did know that I was done deep down but because of the magnitude of what this meant for my future, I wasn't ready to accept it. I wondered how I would ever again feel the ribbon surging through me.

I gathered all my gear, my structure fire turnouts, my axe, my wildland gear and boots, my uniform shirt, pants, and boots, my bedding that I had slept in every night at work, and all the random stuff I had collected over the years and put it in my car.

As I walked back into the apparatus bay, I heard the sound of the engine slowing down Cedar Avenue as it approached the station. The motor of the roll-up door engaged. The *beep beep beep* of the backup alarm sounded as the engine backed into the apparatus bay. Next came the *pphsst* of the parking brake and then came the air-actuated steps coming down as the engine doors were opened. Those sounds were a part of my DNA.

I watched the three-member crew climb out of the engine.

As soon as they saw me, they came over and gave me giant hugs. They'd brought lunch, and we gathered around the familiar table and sat in the familiar chairs, eating. They caught me up on all the department gossip.

After lunch, Wyatt and I talked.

"So how much shit has everyone been talking about me?" I asked.

"No one has been talking shit about you," he said. "Ever since you left, the only thing anyone has said is if this could happen to you, it could happen to any of us."

Hearing this, my brain did a flip and my heart skipped a beat. As usual, I had assumed everyone thought I was a loser. Wyatt's words made me visible . . . made me count.

CHAPTER THIRTY-FIVE

I played in a tennis league where players are sorted into number groups based on skill level. I was a 3.5. The cool kids were the 4.0s and the 4.5s. The 5s carried celebrity status at my tennis club. At the end of a season, players obsessively watched the new ratings. Many based their self-worth on the rating. I was no exception. Lisa was a 4.0, and I feared being left behind by her.

About a week after getting my 3.5 rating, I had a Saturday league tennis match. I desperately wanted to win. In fact, I had it in my mind that I had to win. My rating couldn't afford another loss. In my mind, of course, a lower rating equaled less worthy.

I cheered silently when my opponent walked onto the court. She was short and thin compared to me, and I could hit the crap out of the ball. I expected to win.

She was good. I thought if I hit the ball harder, she wouldn't be able to hit it back, but this led me to making mistakes called "unforced errors."

I have done this with most of my life. When I got a little behind, I pushed harder and faster. In some situations, it gave me an edge. Now it was hurting me.

With each unforced error, my frustration grew. A switch flipped in my head. I glanced over at Lisa, but she had gone off somewhere. I lost it inside. *I am so lame my wife doesn't even want to watch me. I'm not good enough for her. She doesn't love me, and she's more interested in the other matches.*

With those thoughts swirling in my head, my anger reached a boiling point. I smashed my $180 racquet into pieces and threw it at the fence, so packed with anger and frustration I exploded. My opponent won. We shook hands after the match and I gathered up my crap, put my broken racket back in the bag so the fewest people possible could witness my lack of self-control, and walked down the concrete path toward the front of the club.

I am done. I am done with everything and everyone and myself.

Lisa was watching a match at another court. I walked right in front of her. Our eyes met and the look I gave her could have knocked over an old-growth redwood tree.

You are the cause of my feeling like this, I screamed silently. *My losing is your fault. You watching someone else for even a few minutes means you do not care about me. You do not love me. How could you do this to me?*

I kept walking. Behind me, I heard another tennis player ask, "Where are you going?"

Without looking back, I said, "To the bathroom." But I bee-lined straight past the bathroom to the parking lot. I needed to get the hell out of there.

I threw my tennis shit in the trunk and got in my car, but I didn't know where to go.

As I pulled out of the parking lot driveway, with tears in my eyes, anger in my throat and worthlessness in my heart, I decide to head to the Golden Gate Bridge. *I am going to jump off that motherfucker.*

I knew if I looked at my phone and saw that no one had checked on me, I would be devastated, so I turned my phone off.

As I drove across Highway 37, all I could see were the ghosts of people who'd horrifically lost their lives. But after I got to

Highway 101 and headed south, I started thinking of my wife. *She will be so much better off without me. I have been so hard on her.*

Then I started thinking about my niece, Kat. The amazing ten-year-old who I shared such a deep connection. And what about Alexis, her sister? *What am I doing?*

I took a random exit and found a parking lot. I pulled in, put my car in park, and started bawling.

This is fucked. I can't turn this shit off. If I continue to stick around, I will continue to hurt people. If I kill myself, I will hurt people. I just want to disappear. I punched my car door. *Christy, turn around and get your shit together. I really don't want to die; I want the worthlessness to end. I want the ghosts to stop haunting me. I want to stop having nightmares.*

After punching the door, I could barely open my hand. I screamed in my car. My body filled with anger as I knew I had to go home.

I didn't tell Lisa where I had been, and she didn't ask. For a while, I wondered if she even cared.

Five days later, I saw Grace for my regular Thursday appointment. We talked about Saturday and my drive toward the Golden Gate Bridge. The shame in creating so much drama made the incident difficult to talk about. Grace felt it was important Lisa know what happened, and she offered to have us come in together so I could have some support while I told her.

The next day, Lisa and I saw Grace together. Lisa and I sat on the couch in Grace's office. I felt like a child, full of fear and shame and afraid of being abandoned. When Lisa sat down, I sat as close as I could to her, leaning into her, hoping to create an unbreakable connection. She leaned back into me.

Grace spoke first. "Lisa, I'm sure you know we are here because Christy wants to tell you something. I am here to support the both of you . . . to make sure you both feel heard and if either of you have questions or need help as how to move forward."

Lisa and I both nodded.

Tears gathered in Lisa's eyes as I talked. When I finished my story of driving toward the Golden Gate Bridge with plans to kill myself, Grace stayed quiet. Lisa paused for a moment.

She told me she hadn't questioned me that day because she respected my boundaries, but she'd been petrified. When I had not come back after about ten minutes, she knew something was amiss and had gone home, thinking I might be there. When I wasn't there, she called me. When my phone went straight to voice mail, her heart dropped into her stomach.

She then said, "Christy, only you can decide whether to stay here and continue on your journey with me. I wish I could, but I can't make that happen for you. You have to make that decision."

The energy in the room became still and silent. I first heard what she said, and then I felt it. I'd been looking for this answer my entire life. I thought I needed someone to save me. That had been my compass. If no one would save me, I must not be worthy of being saved. But when Lisa said those words, my desperate search for someone to save me finally ended.

I was the one who had to find hope, I realized. I was the one who had to change the dialogue in my head from being worthless to being enough. No one else could save me. I had to save myself. I decided I was going to catch myself when I didn't want to ask for help. I was going to stop myself when I lacked self-compassion.

CHAPTER THIRTY-SIX

My WCPR client group had remained close since the retreat. In the last week of June, Macy, Madison, and I met at the SFO Airport. We'd made a plan to fly to Arizona to meet up with Tom and Terry, then do a road trip to Memphis, where Terry lived.

Macy, Madison, and I had shared our darkest secrets. But at WCPR, we were all contained within boundaries that kept us safe from judgment. Seeing them now for the first time since the retreat presented an exercise in navigating the depth of vulnerability we had experienced together.

During the first hour together in the airport, our bodies were stiff and self-protective, our conversations simple and unrevealing. We loosened a bit once we sat in a row together on the plane. We talked more, and our bodies became animated. In that row, we moved a layer below the surface. We talked about how members of our families were doing and dipped our toes into our frustrations and struggles.

By the time our plane landed in Arizona and Tom picked us up in his king cab truck, we were more comfortable with one another. But it wasn't until we climbed into Tom's air-conditioned truck and back into the containment of being safe and secure, where no one on the outside could see or hear us, that we could exist as we did at WCPR. Now everything felt right and familiar.

We waited there until Terry's plane finally landed, and he climbed in the truck and joined our dome of safety. We were together again.

The next morning, after spending the night at Tom's house, we tossed our suitcases in the bed of Tom's truck and climbed into the cab. Tom drove and Macy rode shotgun. Madison, Terry, and I sat in the back. The three of us took turns sitting in the middle. We'd made life-size cutouts of the faces of the only missing members of the group, Garrett and Greg, so they could be in pictures with us and be a part of the trip.

We were several hours into our trip, somewhere in the desert of New Mexico, when a wave of anxiety spilled over me with no warning or cause.

I was blindsided, but tried to coach myself. Then a flash of light went off in my brain, like I discovered a new connection. I was with my peers and I needed to change how I dealt with this feeling. *Christy, you have to tell someone and quit trying to fight through this alone. Asking for help is a major part you need to change in order to get better. Ask for help. Now.*

I was tentative but found my voice. "Hey, uh, I'm starting to feel shitty, and I've got that 'I need to get out of here feeling.'"

That's all I needed to say. I didn't have to explain why. As Tom's eyes met mine in the rearview mirror, he said, "We all could use a break from the truck anyway."

He took the next exit and drove down an empty, bumpy road until we were a few miles off the freeway. Desert and shrubs lined both sides of the old, rutted, asphalted road. We walked around and explored while making jokes like little kids. I jumped over a fence with a sign that said, "No Trespassing" and a sliver of control rose from my back and straightened my posture. PTSD usually placed a barrier like a tall, electrified fence around me, the danger signs were everywhere, even if I tried to ignore them.

When I controlled where I went and not some fence or sign, I felt stronger and better.

Just being outside in the fresh air began to settle my vibrating brain and body. But what really helped was being seen and heard by some badass first responders who happened to be my friends. Knowing they had my back allowed me to take some control over my life, even for just for a few minutes.

"Okay, I'm ready," I said.

Without another word, everyone piled back into the truck.

The next morning after breakfast at an IHOP, we continued on the road to Memphis. We joked the entire day, shared stories, and laughed till tears squeezed out of our eyes. But about an hour from Memphis, the sky turned dark and so did Terry.

The closer we got to Memphis, the more Terry transformed. He stared out of the window and his face morphed from joy to suffering to anguish. He stopped talking and physically withdrew into the corner of the back seat. I noticed he seemed to be holding his breath, as if bracing for a punch to the stomach.

When we crossed into Memphis, Terry did what all of us first responders did when we're in the city we worked. From his deflated body, he pointed out places where he responded to shitty calls.

"I was shot at in that parking lot over there."

"I pulled a dead kid out of a car that was on fire in that intersection."

As he talked, he stared out the window, never looking away, as if he watched the call happen. He compressed and hardened, so if anything hit him, it would just bounce off. He shut down.

He soon stopped talking. Watching Terry was like holding up a mirror. We could see in him what PTSD had done to all of us.

Compassion welled inside me as I witnessed Terry's transformation. I wanted to take his pain away. The rest of us never talked about it, but I knew we all felt in that moment how hard we'd been on ourselves through this journey with PTSD.

Terry needed love, patience, and compassion from us. I knew I needed to offer those very things to myself. Easier said than done.

CHAPTER THIRTY-SEVEN

I drove up to Oregon to visit my dad in the fall. He and Barbara lived out in the mountains in a cozy cabin he'd built himself.

I visited my dad only a few times a year. Sometimes our relationship was strained because of my resentments from childhood, but things between us had improved. He and my stepmom always made me feel welcome. Their love brought me safety and security.

My dad called me a few days before I left for the drive up to discuss the menu. He told me he'd planned all my family favorites: Grandma's stuffed flank steak, his tacos, his spaghetti with as much garlic bread as one can eat, Great-Grandpa's "baby poop soup," and green cheese and peanut butter toast. The best comfort food ever.

When I first arrived, Barbara was eager to show me to the giant batch of chocolate chip cookies she'd made for me. I knew what was in store—we'd spend a lot of time eating, playing cribbage, drinking high-balls, and watching their favorite science fiction movies. I was right where I needed to be.

At WCPR and with Grace, everyone spoke of the power of vulnerability. To be genuine and not live in fear, I learned that being vulnerable was a strength not a weakness. My dad had transformed into someone I knew I could count on, someone who would lovingly take care of me when I needed help. After everything I'd gone through, I had an urge to sit on my dad's lap and have him hold me. I couldn't remember either of my parents ever having held me over the years.

Throughout the visit with him, I pictured sitting on his lap in my mind, but I was too afraid to ask and be rejected. But one evening, as I sat on the couch and he sat in his chair, something inside of me yelled, *Go for it now!*

I got up from the couch and took a few steps until I stood in front of him.

"I want to sit in your lap," I said, nervously.

"Okay," he replied, with uncertainty in his voice.

As I carefully sat down, we laughed at the awkwardness of my size trying to fit in his lap. I leaned my head against his shoulder, and he put his arms around me.

After a few minutes, I said, "Tell me when your legs go numb, and I will get up."

"My legs are just fine," he said.

CHAPTER THIRTY-EIGHT

Every morning as I drove to work in Berkeley, I'd pass through the Caldecott Tunnel. As I crested the top of Tunnel Avenue, I could see the island of Alcatraz. On the engine, as we drove down Alcatraz Avenue, the view of the infamous prison stood out even more. Occasionally, I'd mention how kick-ass it would be to make that swim. In the past year, I had attended the WCPR retreat, gone to the Grand Canyon, driven across the country with my amazing PTSD cohorts, and had a significant visit with my dad.

I wanted a challenge, and the swim popped in my mind. It would summon and control my ribbon. The longer I went without my ribbon, the stronger the pull became. I opened my laptop and googled the swim.

The Sharkfest Escape from Alcatraz Swim was happening on August 13, a full ten months away. I registered.

Lisa walked into the room minutes later.

"I just signed up for the Alcatraz swim!" I told her.

With a straight face and sarcastic voice, she said, "That's a great idea, especially since you hate to swim."

Lisa was correct. I didn't like to swim, but not because of the water. Since my teenage years, I hadn't been comfortable in my body in public. I didn't look like the other girls in school, who had pretty, long hair and a never-ending supply of nice clothes. My hair was thick as fishing line, and I had a ton of it.

Puberty delivered big, uncomfortable boobs, which I hated. And although my DNA was only 34% Italian, somehow I got 100% of the dark-thick-hair-everywhere gene.

As I got older, I'd get waxed, but that in-between stage looked dreadful in a bathing suit. I was sure everyone at the pool would stare at me and think, "Wow, she looks disgusting in that suit."

If I was going to complete the Alcatraz swim, I'd have to train by swimming countless hours in a public pool, while wearing a bathing suit. I wasn't going to let my fear keep me from completing that swim.

I'm doing this.

A couple days later, I asked my friend Darcy, a swimmer, to take me bathing suit shopping. I asked Darcy because Lisa doesn't swim. She doesn't even own a bathing suit. Darcy and I pulled into the parking lot of Sports Basement and my insides rebelled. This was a bad idea. I would have preferred to run into a burning building than try on a bathing suit. But Darcy would never think less of me, and she would be honest.

She helped me pick out some suits. After struggling into one, I opened the door and Darcy quickly said, "Oh my God no!" and we both laughed.

In the end, I decided on a men's swimsuit—long, form-fitting shorts—and a plain sports bra.

I stood in front of Darcy with my arms out and my body saying, *Well here I am.* "If you didn't know me and saw me at the pool, what would you think?"

She put her hands on her hips and said, "If I saw you at the pool, I'd say there goes a swimmer."

Just the words I needed to hear.

In the water, gravity released its pull, leaving me suspended. Every burden and load that sat on my shoulders lost its heaviness under the surface. Movements became slow and deliberate. When space around me filled with water, I became part of it. I couldn't fall or run away. Noise became muffled and slow.

The serenity of the water pulled at me. I wanted to be in the water as much as possible. I swam laps for about an hour, then went to the deep diving well to just 'be' in the water. I floated on my back and closed my eyes. I sank far under the water and stayed suspended for as long as I could, gently holding my breath. I had found the peace I'd been searching for.

CHAPTER THIRTY-NINE

In the middle of the second period of a hockey game in December, the inside of my left butt check screamed at me in pain. I already wasn't playing well. I was slow, my passes were missing their target, and I couldn't catch a pass. I endlessly apologized to my team.

I made self-deprecating jokes instead of engaging silently in my usual relentless attack on myself about how bad I sucked and didn't deserve to be there. Not a model of good self-esteem, but it was progress.

I was supposed to play in a second game. I approached the team captain and asked, "Hey Shauna, do you have enough players for your game? I did something to my hip, and I don't think I should play."

Shauna laced up her skate and said, "We can play with nine. Don't even worry about it."

Normally the minimum is ten. I hesitated for a moment, waiting for my inner critic to berate me. Something had shifted in my head. There was quiet. I did not beat myself up mercilessly for being weak. Instead, I just changed out of my gear and into dry clothes.

I slung my hockey bag over my shoulder, and it seemed to weigh eight thousand pounds. A couple of people offered to carry my bag out, but I wouldn't let them—I hadn't come that far in self-care yet. I made the hour drive home, left everything in my car and hobbled into the house.

I had broken each of my legs, and I had crushed my finger with a sledgehammer. But this pain intertwined with every part of my body. I felt pain when I moved, and I felt pain when I remained still. This was a close-your-eyes-and-grit-your-teeth pain

What the hell is going on?

Since it was December and so close to Christmas, the earliest I could get in to see an orthopedic doctor was the end of January.

Over the next few days, Lisa and my friends badgered me. "Go to the emergency room!"

The pain worsened and I finally listened to them.

In the waiting room, sitting hurt like hell. I wanted to lie on the floor, but luckily, they called my name before I succumbed. A young doctor wearing dark-blue scrubs with his name embroidered in white cursive came in and asked a few questions.

"I see your leg is spasming quite a bit," he noted. "Does that bother you?"

His question confirmed my thoughts about coming here. All I got was a bill, a prescription for a weak anti-inflammatory, a lame Toradol shot in my other butt cheek, and an X-ray. I was informed they may or may not follow up with the results.

I got home and marched right back into bed in agony and tears. I felt beaten and useless. I couldn't believe the ineptitude and uselessness of that doctor.

The month that followed was difficult. I was in too much pain to help with cooking or cleaning at Christmas. Not working out caused me to be irritable even without my PTSD. But I strove to change the dialogue in my head, and consciously chose acceptance. It worked.

Before, I would have spent the entire month being miserable. I'd be mad at myself for not being able to pull my own weight, uncomfortable accepting help from those around me.

Now, even though it wasn't easy, I was able to accept the needed help and understood asking didn't make me a weak person.

After finally getting a hip MRI in late January, I drove to Oakland to discuss the results with a new doctor.

He squished his face up and rubbed his chin. "You have a torn labrum. I am just not convinced that your pain isn't being caused by something else. Let me see you do a squat."

My eyes widened. "You want me to do a squat?"

"Yes, please."

I slid off the examination table, dragging with me the crunchy paper that was stuck to the back of my leg. I held onto the table and very slowly and carefully did a squat. The movement was excruciating.

The doc squished up his face again and said, "All right. Let's do surgery and get a look. Okay?"

He said this as if he'd just lost an argument. I hated the idea of surgery, but I couldn't take the pain in my hip anymore.

"Okay," I said. "Please just make the pain stop."

I finally got my hip fixed on March 31, 2016, three months after the intense pain had started.

When my surgeon came by the recovery room after the procedure was done, he informed me that there was significantly more damage than he'd expected. "The labrum was torn and then had a compound tear," he explained. "It was twisted and stuck in the joint. That kind of damage is usually only something we see with significant trauma."

"Don't you now feel bad for making me do a squat?"

"Yes, yes I do," he smiled.

I was relieved to be on the mend. But once I was back at home, I felt stuck. I worried about my Alcatraz swim. The only place I felt physically comfortable was in a recliner—but mentally I wanted to be back in the water.

It took about two weeks of worrying before a flash of light went off in my head, and I realized something I should have known already. I would not be stuck forever. I would not be disconnected from everything and everyone forever.

Grace often told me, "Take each day as it comes, and cherish yourself in it."

I decided to listen to her.

CHAPTER FORTY

About a month after my surgery, I had an appointment with Grace. I parked my car under the large oak trees surrounding her office. A quick look at my phone before I got out of my car revealed a call from my department's deputy chief. She didn't leave a message, and I knew why. I was being retired, or as Berkeley called it, "separated from the city."

I immediately called her back, and it went straight to voicemail. I left a quick message and only had five minutes until my appointment, so I shot her a text. "Hey, I just tried calling your desk, but now I can't talk. Am I being taken off the books? I know it's better to talk about it in person, but with the timing right now, it would be good to know."

I opened the door of the building and pleaded in my head, *Please, Chief, respond. I don't want to spend the next hour talking about "what if." I have been "what if'ing" for the last year, and I can't take it anymore.*

I'd known this was coming, but I'd kept the possibility open that I could go back. It's like when my beloved grandpa died from a long battle with cancer. Toward the end, I knew he was going to die and hoped it would come soon to relieve his suffering. When he died, I was shocked and wanted to scream, *Wait! I didn't mean this!!* The finality didn't come until it was over.

I walked into the waiting room and sat in my usual chair.

Finally, a text came through., "Sorry! I didn't recognize your number. Thanks for your second text. Yes, you are separated effective March 22."

I wrote back a quick, "Thank you for letting me know." When I hit "send," the door opened, and Grace's warm smile appeared. How grateful I was for her smile.

I settled into her office, grabbed a pillow to hold onto, and shared what had just transpired. We spent the entire session talking about how I was no longer a firefighter. Now, when people asked me what I did, I'd have to say, "I was a firefighter."

The difference between "was" and "am" is a big deal. A person who is a firefighter is important, purposeful, self-sufficient, and belongs. Kids want to be you. Adults are amazed by you. The leap is extraordinary, going from being a member of the sworn personnel to being a regular "citizen." Prior to this journey, I would have fought, argued, been pissed off, and gone into isolation. But with everything I learned and the tools I had gained, I could put a name to losing my job. Grief. And with a name, I could deal with it by acknowledging my loss, talking about it, and yes, even crying, knowing "why" I was crying.

A few days later, a letter arrived from the City of Berkeley.

April 12, 2016

Dear Mr. Warren:

Pursuant to the authority delegated to me by action of the City Council of the City of Berkeley, I hereby determine that Christine E. Warren, a local safety member, employed by the agency, is incapacitated for performance of her duties in the position of Fire Captain II.

She is not able to return to her previous duties as a firefighter and fire captain. She is precluded from responding to fires and medical emergencies, supervising and training firefighters, and handling high-stress emergency responses, which involve dangerous or life-threatening incidents, serious injury, or death.

"Mr. Warren" is not a typo on my part. The notification letter of my separation was addressed to Mr. Warren. Unbelievable. It also included other legal and employment jargon. I was thankful the deputy chief had called me and not just left me to receive this impersonal letter with its ridiculous typo. This felt like a breakup—like Berkeley was dumping me. I knew at some point the breakup was coming. I had already relinquished my desire to fight or "fix" myself in order to get my job back. Relieved I didn't have to question whether to go back to work or retire, I still couldn't take in the entirety of what this meant. I'd have to let go in small pieces.

CHAPTER FORTY-ONE

At my eight-week post-surgery checkup, I sat on the examination table with the crinkly paper on top. My hip had been feeling great, and I'd been swimming a lot. I'd bought a wetsuit for the Alcatraz swim and couldn't wait for the race.

The obligatory knock came at the door, and my handsome surgeon walked in wearing a pair of green hospital scrubs.

"How's the hip?" he asked.

"It's good! I said. "I've been swimming a lot and am going to do the Escape from Alcatraz swim next month."

"No, you aren't," he said firmly. "Your hip isn't ready for open-water swimming."

"Are you serious?"

"I told you this was going to take a year."

Another carpet ripped out from under me. Would I ever get a break?

Instead of jumping off of a ferry into the cold bay and escaping Alcatraz, for the next month I aimlessly wandered around in circles wondering who, what, where, how, and why in the hell I was.

"You are not lost. You are in transition," Grace told me.

But I had lost my job—and with it, access to my ribbon. My hypervigilance increased as I looked for any situation around me where I could wrestle with my ribbon. I searched for someone's house to catch fire, a bad car wreck—anything that would summon the ribbon. But nothing worked. Swimming brought me peace, but not the surge of electricity I craved.

Eventually, though, I started listening to Grace, and I realized she was right. I was in transition. I was learning to separate shame from not being able to do my job. And I wanted to share my journey, and the lessons I'd learned, with my former colleagues.

I'd left work on October 6, 2014, and I'd never come back. No one really knew what happened, I just disappeared. I felt strong and safe enough now to let my friends and coworkers know. I also wanted to share what I'd been through in case anyone else was suffering. I did not want anyone to go through what I went through alone.

I wrote an email and sent it to the entire department.

My dear BFD brothers and sisters,

First of all, it is difficult to describe how much I miss everyone and how much I miss my job. Not having to get up in the middle of the night is amazing, but I really loved that job.

I think most of you know why I left so hastily. I was diagnosed with PTSD and if I stayed any longer, it was most likely going to kill me. I don't say that lightly. I fought it for almost a year before I finally turned in my paperwork to go off. I had every intention of coming back. I got off duty the morning of October 6 and disappeared because I didn't know what was happening to me. I was so full of shame. I know I have been really hard on many of you, and I always tried to be perfect. (I know I wasn't even close.) When I had to leave, I felt like such a hypocrite. I was so ashamed and felt like a total failure.

I will say that every phone call, text, and FB message I got meant the world to me, especially because I could be such an asshole. I apologize for most of the times I was an asshole, and I mean this sincerely.

I am finally doing much better. I have learned that PTSD is actually a physiological brain injury and not a weakness. If any of you are feeling any symptoms, please get help before it consumes you. And by the way, alcohol makes it worse. I know from experience.

The number of firefighter suicides have been increasing every year. If anyone needs anything else, please do not hesitate to contact me, especially if you need someone to talk to regarding PTSD stuff or crappy call stuff or anything. I don't want anyone to go through this crap alone.

And if you are someone who is struggling right now, you aren't alone. Besides the one year waiting list to get into WCPR, there are one hundred and fifty firefighters from Chicago fire who are trying to get to the WCPR retreat.

I really miss you guys. Please be safe and take care of yourselves.

Christy

Sending the letter off to the department gave me some relief and empowerment. I received some thoughtful emails in response, which validated me—but that validation quickly wore off.

Grace said I was still grieving. It wasn't just my job I'd lost, but also my identity, value, purpose, family, and belonging.

For a while I stood on the outside alone, lost, devalued, not sure of who I was or supposed to be. But eventually, I got sick of wandering around, feeling lost, and wanting my job back. I wanted to move forward, to find purpose again.

After being on meds for a while, I had greater control of my mind. It no longer spun out of control, taking me back through all the years of death and dying. From time to time, the PTSD would still try to drag me back down into its depths, but now I knew how to fight back and stop it.

Identifying the problem was the first step. Instead of remaining stuck and bemoaning what I'd lost, acknowledging the loss and accepting there was nothing to do but move forward gave me a map for how to get my life back—something worth celebrating.

CHAPTER FORTY-TWO

O ne evening, a week after I emailed the department, my cell phone rang, and I actually answered it.

"Hey, Christy. This is Marc."

"Marc! How are you?" Marc was a firefighter I'd worked with in Berkeley.

"Um. Not so good. Now you don't have to tell me any of your personal business, but I have PTSD."

"Oh, I am so sorry. I am so sorry you're going through this. Please know you're not alone, and we'll get you through this."

Marc and I talked for a while. He talked about all the PTSD symptoms he was having and how he just couldn't take it anymore. He shared with me he felt suicidal. "I carry a single bullet with me everywhere I go," he said. "I obsess over this bullet and spend every day working to keep from putting it into my head."

"The first thing you need to do is call my friend Luke," I said. "Luke is with WCPR. Even if you don't think you need to go, call and get yourself on the wait list. And please Marc, call me anytime you need anything."

Marc sent me a text the next day telling me he got his name on the waiting list to get into WCPR. I was thankful he had made the call.

Not long after my conversation with Marc, the Berkeley Fire-fighters Association, our union, put together a peer counseling team. Julian, the guy heading it up, reached out to me and asked if I would share my story with him. We sat across from each other. As I talked and shared my story, he feverishly wrote in a notebook and said, "Wow" a lot. We sat at the table and talked for about an hour and a half.

By the middle of September, the eight members of the BFD Peer Counseling Unit (PCU) were ready to roll out the program to the department. They held educational sessions explaining everything about the PCU. They asked me and Marc if we would be willing to share our story with everyone during these sessions.

Of course, we agreed to. We both never wanted anyone to go through what we had alone.

The classroom at the training center smelled like paper and burned coffee, which I remembered from my training days. Marc and I had decided he would go first, so I sat in the back corner and listened to the rumbling of the truck and fire engines arrive and back into the drill grounds, while Marc leaned against the podium in the front of the classroom, tumbling a single bullet between his fingers.

The department had three shifts—the A, B, and C shifts. The A shift worked forty-eight hours; the B shift worked forty-eight hours; and the C shift worked forty-eight hours. Then it started all over again with the A shift. To get the entire department to attend a training, each shift had to send half the department to attend and the other half to cover the city. So, Marc and I would tell our story six times.

We shared our stories with the first group. Everyone responded with care, concern, and understanding. I did not feel judgment from anyone. I cut loose a heavy weight I'd been dragging behind me.

But telling my story had another effect, too. Each time I told my story, losing my job became more real. The realization sank deeper that I would never put on my uniform, climb into an engine, and head back out into the streets ever again. This PTSD bullshit had robbed me of my full career. I missed being at the station. I missed how comfortable my turnout pants were (except on a warm day). I missed warm evenings riding in the engine with the windows down. I missed everything in the engine cab smelling like smoke. I did not miss being exhausted all the time, but I did miss being exhausted after working my ass off doing something good. I missed the crazy calls and all the different people I met. I missed driving the tiller on the truck. I missed hearing and feeling the force of the 470 horsepower engine. I missed my morning cup of coffee on the second day of a forty-eight-hour shift. We'd sit around the table with our hair fucked up and wearing what we had slept in, just like being at home with our families.

The hardest shift to share with was, of course, the B shift, my old shift. These were the people I had consistently worked with, ate with, and brushed my teeth with. I fought fires with them and saved and lost lives with them.

I told them when it first started and how I didn't know what was happening to me. I told them how hard I fought to keep anyone from knowing, from having any idea a swollen river of anxiety and panic raged inside of me every time the tones went off. I told them how being haunted by calls felt like being trapped in a movie theater and having to watch horrible images over and over because my eyes would not close. I told them how I refused to take meds because I felt I should be able to do it by myself and the shame I experienced taking psychiatric meds. Then I told them how the medications saved me. I told them alcohol, which most people in the room used, wouldn't fix it.

"I tried," I told them. "It doesn't work."

I decided to go to one of my favorite taco places in Berkeley, Gordo's, on my way home for some lunch. As soon as I found a parking space around the corner from Gordo's and started walking toward College Ave, a fire engine siren screamed from the south from the direction of Oakland. As it sped through the intersection, I saw it was an Oakland engine. Oakland Fire would only be dispatched into Berkeley if a large incident had occurred.

I turned the corner onto College Avenue and walked north. I saw about a half mile down the street, thick gray smoke billowed into and across the street. Lots of it.

In the millisecond I saw the smoke, my chest felt as though it has been hit with a sledgehammer. My body reeled backward, yet still had forward momentum, going toward the smoke. I almost fell to the ground because parts of my body tried to turn around and run away and the other parts tried to run toward the smoke.

My response was visceral, *Hurry and get there and do what I can to help. Catch a hydrant, pull some hose, whatever needs doing outside the building.* No question existed in my mind that I should go. But my nervous system gripped every muscle I possessed and took flight.

I ran back to my 4Runner and escaped into my vehicle. In an instant, being hungry or the idea of going to Gordo's evaporated from my mind. I breathed as though I had just run up a long, steep hill as fast as I could. I drove away like a snarling rabid wolf nipped at the backs of my legs.

Shame began to swell and snowball inside of me until tears streamed down my face. *Who or what kind of person worthy to be a firefighter runs away? Real firefighters run toward danger, not away. My shift, my peers, people I cared about, ran into that fire.*

I fucking ran away.

If there were such a thing as a chasm of disgrace, I ended up at the bottom.

I may have been retired, but once a firefighter, always a firefighter. Even though I had lost my identity as a firefighter, I still had it in my heart and body. After running away from that fire, and as I struggled to figure out who I was, I had just proved I didn't have the fighter heart anymore.

Who in the hell am I now?

Less than two weeks after the incident, I headed back up to WCPR. I looked forward to talking about what had happened and help rid the shame I'd wrapped around me like plastic wrap.

As the start of the retreat came closer, I became more nervous. My nerves continued to tap at me all over my body until Monday, when we did a peer debriefing.

During the debriefing, I talked about the devastation I had experienced when I ran away from the fire last month. I cried and just as I had hoped, my peers' reactions helped me peel off the suffocating plastic wrap.

Once I shed my shame, I concentrated on moving forward and working on what I needed to do to recover from all of what was happening to me. I told myself I was in recovery from a brain injury. I was also recovering from a hip injury. A brain injury had caused me to run away from the smoke and fire; nothing in my heart had ever changed. I put all my energy toward getting better, not being pissed off and stuck all the time.

I reminded myself what Grace would tell me and would repeat this to myself. *I am an adult. I am going to be fine. I am worthy. I have control over myself! I choose to feel shitty. Concentrate on me and only me. Do what makes me happy. Forget the bad and focus on the good. I can only take care of me. I belong here, wherever that is and wherever I am, I belong right there. I am enough. I am worthy.*

I had to keep telling myself this, but the more I did it, the closer I came to believing it.

It was time for the BFD's annual retirement dinner in April. I was to be one of the honorees. I was nervous. Not making it to "retirement" had been a vast source of shame for me. I didn't make it to fifty, which meant to me that I wasn't retiring honorably. I was convinced I'd have to face that perception from others at the dinner. Instead, I heard genuine happy congratulations. Not one person said "sorry" or "too bad" or "well, you tried." One coworker told me he was scared shitless that what happened to me could happen to him.

When we sat down for dinner, I made sure I sat next to my former battalion chief who I had spent the early part and biggest bulk of my career with. When we were finished eating, I turned my chair to face him directly.

I said, "Chief, I just want to apologize for being so hard on you. You were always so good to me, and I constantly complained you didn't do enough."

He said, "You weren't that hard on me. I wanted my shift to be the best shift in the department. So it was no accident you were on my shift. I put you on it."

Quietly, I took in what he had said. My goal in the fire service was to be a mighty enough firefighter so people would want me on their crew. I said, "That really means a lot to me. I still want you to know I am sorry for all the angst I caused. I cannot tell you how much I appreciate the guidance, knowledge, and patience you showed me."

The guys from Station 2 had invited me to dinner a handful of times since I had left. At first, I was honest with them and said I'll come when I'm ready. Then the time came when I thought I should be ready, and I'd make a date. Then just prior to the date, I'd make up a reason why I couldn't go.

Finally, we made a date I promised myself I would stick to. I finally felt ready—until the day came. My body was caught in a tug-o-war of fight or flight. I slipped two Ativan in my pocket, just in case. Of course, the traffic sucked, so it just prolonged and intensified my anxiety.

The best route to Station 2 was through Engine 3's district, the road through fraternity row and down Bancroft. As I drove by the fraternity houses, my anxiety melted away. Every single fraternity on this long street had caused me and my crews so much angst. I had responded to calls at each one countless times. Knowing I never had to deal with these shitheads and their bullshit ever again, I smiled.

When I arrived at Station 2, nothing had changed except two new guys. One of my favorite guys, Bobby Law, sat in a recliner watching YouTube videos of stuff being destroyed by a hydraulic press. I jumped on him and received a big hug. I got more hugs from the guys and a couple of strong handshakes from the two new kids. We joked and gave each other shit, just like I'd never left.

At dinner we talked about funny past calls and had some good belly laughs. They updated me on the regulars (the people who would call 911 all the time) . . . who had died and how the survivors were doing. They brought me up to date on department gossip. In the space between the kitchen and dining area, there was a large support post where Berkeley fire members signed their name and hire date. I found my signature and thought, *I do still belong.* I might be retired, but I'd always be a part of this department.

My body and brain had braced themselves for the sounds and actions of getting a call. *If it happens, will I start crying? Will anxiety take over my body, causing me to feel like I have to get the hell out of here?*

Then the moment I'd been anxiously anticipating arrived. A call came in for the engine and the ambulance. My preparation helped. I did not panic nor experience any anxiety. I counted it as a win for the day.

The engine came back and then had to leave again. The sounds and routines were still live in my being. I could have easily picked up right where I left off and taken those easy calls without missing a beat. But when that bad call came, I knew I would have taken fifty-five steps backward in my recovery.

I left the station around 8:00 p.m., when everyone in the department usually tries to wind down and get some time to themselves—to call home, go to their bunks, finish up paperwork, and to bring closure to the day. But now I was a guest, and I was leaving the station to go home.

Leaving felt okay. I didn't leave sad or angry. I was relieved I could go home and crawl into bed with my wife and stay there all night. Those guys I just left would be getting up at all hours of the night to answer calls for help. However, they didn't see me as a failure. They saw me as someone who'd gotten seriously injured on the job and was thankful to be alive.

And I was.

CHAPTER FORTY-THREE

At 4:30 a.m. on June 4, 2017, I reached my arm out from under the covers and my hand patted around my nightstand, searching for the spot on my iPhone to shut off the alarm and stop the music of the Masked Intruders yelling at me to "Stick 'em Up."

Some part of my hand finally found the spot, and the music stopped.

I lay there for another ten minutes. Without opening her eyes, Lisa said, "Are we changing our mind?"

I sat up with my legs off the bed and said, "Hell, no." I slowly stood up and lumbered to the kitchen for a glass of water.

As I drank my water, I thought, *Jumping off a perfectly good boat into the freezing cold bay and swimming for a mile and a half sounds like a horrible idea.* I went to the bathroom and almost fell asleep on the toilet.

I'd left myself little time to get out of the house, so I could sleep every available minute. The night before, I had packed my bag with my wetsuit, goggles, ear plugs, towels, and dry underpants and set it by the front door. Lisa got up shortly after me. She was ready to go shortly after me. We stopped for coffee, then picked up my dad from the hotel where he and my stepmom were staying. It was still dark when he climbed in the car to start the thirty-minute drive to San Francisco.

As we drove over the Bay Bridge, the sun began its daily rise from the east. I stayed on the right side of the bridge so I could see Alcatraz. From the view of the bridge, the space between the island and the shore loomed large. It was a long way to swim. We wove through the city and made our way to Aquatic Park.

It was a gorgeous day in San Francisco, perfect for the experience—a cloudless sky and a light, cool breeze. The bay did not resemble the stories I'd heard of treacherous currents and choppy water, an angry sea reminiscent of a Greek novel in which the gods were furious. Instead, the water was calm (the Greek Gods must have been asleep), the sun was shining, and the air was still. Early risers walked their dogs or just themselves along the shore walkway. The small beach and the cement bleachers began filling with people putting on wetsuits.

I checked in, then wedged my body into my black-and-pink neoprene suit and my head into the yellow swim cap. I handed my backpack off to Lisa, gave her a kiss and my dad a hug, and walked with a thousand upright seals with yellow heads down Jefferson Street toward the ferries, my heart swelling with excitement.

Although hundreds of people surrounded me, I felt alone on this journey. I was torn between wanting to appear like I knew what I was doing and to be fully open and present. To be fully present, I had to allow in the vulnerability of doing this for the first time in my life.

I walked in the front of the line of people heading toward the ferry. I'd been given some advice prior, where slower swimmers should be the first to be in the water. I stepped off to the side and let people go ahead of me. The first people on the ferries would be the last ones off.

When we arrived at the loading dock, the race director yelled race instructions, but I couldn't hear what he said. I had read about this swim. "Make sure you pay close attention to the morning race instructions."

He continued to yell the instructions several more times. We were to follow the boat with the giant orange balls on it. Thankfully, it would not be a problem for me.

I was one of the last to board the ferry. A few hundred people in wetsuits and a few in bathing suits milled around the large, open space. I found a seat next to the open door I would jump out of and enjoyed the ride.

Jumping off the ferry brought me back to being a kid, when the only thing I liked about swimming was jumping into the pool. I was the third person to jump off the ferry, and I performed a beautiful cannon ball. Jumping in with legs straight meant I would submerge and take longer to get back up to the surface. The longer I lingered in the water right off the boat, the greater my chances of someone jumping on top of me. I quickly surfaced and swam away about fifty meters. I was in the middle of the bay! People poured out of the ferries into the water. I swam toward the mass of kayakers, which marked the starting line. I still hadn't noticed the cold of the water.

About hundred meters ahead of the starting line, ten San Francisco cops on jet skis spun doughnuts in the water. From somewhere, I heard music playing. There were boats, kayaks, and paddle boarders scattered over an area the size of a football field. Being out there was like being alone at a giant party, but I didn't sulk. I was eager to join in and become a part of the celebration. I did not care about being a novice or feeling out of place. I had not been this happy in a long time.

Suddenly, the mass of yellow heads lurched forward and started to swim. I hadn't even heard the starting horn. The boat with the orange balls began to motor. Following after it, I felt like a rabbit being led around by a giant, round carrot.

I stopped a few times during the swim to catch my breath and glance at the incredible scenery. My eyes sitting only a few inches above the water in such an enormous expanse of openness made me become part of the earth just like the Grand Canyon. Instead of worrying about how fast I could swim, I indulged in this experience. I could see the Golden Gate Bridge, the Bay Bridge, and the San Francisco skyline. I always made sure there were people behind me, because as important as "stopping to smell the roses" was, not finishing last was more important. Second to last, okay, but not last.

I entered the small opening of Aquatic Park. *Holy shit, I am going to make it!* I stopped swimming and searched for the finish chute on the beach. I looked for a couple of blue panels on the beach, but they were difficult to find in the large crowd of people. Finally, I found it and started swimming toward it.

Time to impress the fans, I thought. I put my face back in the cold water and shifted my swim engine to turbo.

After a few minutes, I lifted my head to take a quick look and could not see a single person. I stopped swimming to find out where in the hell I was and realized the current had carried me so far to the left that I was completely off course. I said a few expletives to myself, reoriented my body, and turned the speed on again. *I am really moving now! Fuck ya!*

I looked up again, and for a second time, everyone had disappeared. *I turned left! Again!*

This happened a third time before I finally got it right. As I got closer to the beach, fatigued from my hard-charging left detours, I thought the water was shallow enough to touch the bottom and walk out. I orienteded my body vertically and stretched my legs to touch sand beneath my feet. Nope.

Arghh! I had to get horizontal again and swim. I just wanted to stand up and walk.

I swam a little farther, and finally, my feet touched bottom and I walked out of the water.

The second I stepped onto the beach, I heard my name. My amazing friends Julie, Cathie, and Sharlene had come from Gilroy to watch me finish. They'd even made awesome signs. I wanted to run and hug them, but I was too busy being ushered through the finish chute by volunteers.

As I trotted through the chute, basking in my awesome glow, I saw my time: 52:33. Way under the allotted time.

Right after the finish line, Lisa's eyes met mine with a matching smile. A few steps later, she was right in front of me and I gave her a giant, wet hug, beaming from ear to ear.

There is that overused cliché, which said, "When one door closes, another one opens." For me, when PTSD closed the door to one of the most important parts of me, I believed I'd been shut off from who I was. I believed I would not, and could not, survive. I'd walked through that door every day of my life since I was nineteen. Once it slammed shut in my face, I stood in the cold, lonely hallway, unable to open the door leading to a purpose. The purpose gave me opportunity to harness the ribbon that gave me clarity and meaning, the ribbon that took away my worry, doubt, pain, and sense of worthlessness.

In the hallway, I had pounded on the door, praying it would open. But it didn't. The hallway had filled with unbearable noise and the blackest darkness. As I took a few steps back from the door to build up speed to plow through the door, I fell into a deep hole.

At the bottom of the hole, I stewed in my anger, alone, until one day someone or something or the universe or God dropped a note into the pit. The note slowly fell, wafting down, until I grabbed the small square piece of paper out of the air. The word "Hope" was written on it.

I finally screamed, "Help!" sure no one would come. But amazing people came and stood around the hole. They dropped a rope and taught me how to climb out. They led me to a different hallway full of light, quietness, and new doors.

It took a while, but I started to try those new doors. They led me to wonderful things, but I still feared the ribbon was lost forever.

But as I stood on the ferry before my swim, waiting to jump, the ribbon had swirled inside me. Not as fast and hot as before, but it was there. My body had mastered the ribbon, and I jumped out of the ferry and into the cold water of the San Francisco Bay. Clarity and presence permeated my mind and body while I swam to shore.

EPILOGUE

Being invisible as a kid left an unbearably painful hole in the middle of my heart. The only way to escape the pain was to never look at it, feel it, or acknowledge it. The only way I knew how to escape it was to run away from it, cover it so no one could see it. I poured myself into a job that entailed saving others, fixing their problems so I never had to face my own.

People would ask me, "My goodness, how do you run into a burning building?"

But it was easy when I was being chased by something more dangerous than a large wooden box on fire—my own demons.

I don't run anymore. Nothing is chasing me.

When asked what Lisa wanted to do when I got off work, she would say, "It depends on what walks through the front door in the morning."

I always thought she was referring to how much sleep I got. I now realized what she really meant. Which Christy would come home? The one who just responded to a horrible car accident and came home distant and distracted? Or the one who had to deal with a kid who was severely injured due to lack of supervision or parenting? For years my wife endured this.

To come out the other side of PTSD, I had to walk into and through my unhealed wounds. PTSD stole my self-worth, leaving me to reclaim it bit by bit, working hard to allow my

271

worthiness to refill me. I had to open and expose my heart and let vulnerability in. PTSD was a physical, biological brain injury, which screwed with every part of my being. Survivors are strong motherfuckers.

Experts told me PTSD never completely went away, but it would get to the point where it became hardly noticeable.

Today, I still have to manage my injury. I still take medications. I still see my psychiatrist and therapist, although less frequently. A few times a month I still wake up in a cold sweat and scream from a nightmare. Images from calls still pop into my consciousness occasionally. But I am not haunted anymore. None of it ruins my day. I sometimes still get triggered. When that happens, I immediately identify what's going on, work through it, and then go about my day. I don't berate myself asking, *How in the hell did I get here? How did I let this PTSD bullshit happen?!* Instead, I remind myself, *Wow! Look where I am! I am happy and calm and safe.*

And how did I get here? Hard work, making healthy choices, and medication. I also had people around me who loved me and stuck with me—my wife in particular. I changed the dialogue in my head and held onto the idea of hope, even when I had none.

The crushing grip PTSD holds around your neck will not last forever.

I am here to say, it won't.

ACKNOWLEDGMENTS

I rarely read the acknowledgment pages of a book. Unless, of course, it's a really good book that I don't want to end. Then I will read every single word, of every single page. But now that I know just how many people it takes to get a book into the reader's hands, I make sure I take the time to read them.

There are so many people to thank.

First, to my wife, Lisa, who read everything I wrote and gave me not only the courage to continue writing my book, but the courage to keep on living. There are no words to express my love for you and thank you for putting up with me and us.

Thank you Tiara Inserto, an author herself, for being the very first person to read a very shitty half-completed, first rough draft. When we sat down in your kitchen to talk about my manuscript, you wrapped your arms around it and pulled it into your chest and said, "I *love* this." Your belief gave me permission to believe.

I owe my happiness and life to all of the founders of WCPR, for building your dream to save our lives. And specifically, thank you to the WCPR staff of Session 114—Mark Kamena, Dian Barkan, Sue Faria, Barb, Big Joe, Nick, Fireman Bob, and my six cohorts—you all directly saved my life.

Thank you to Yvonne, who never left my side no matter how difficult I could be. I can't even find the words to describe what you meant to me and my recovery. The love and grace that you gave me from the center of your heart sustained me through all my darkest times.

Thank you, Kelly Sommerset, who kept me moving when I would get stuck.

Thank you, Linda Brown. Oh Linda Brown, to have you fight for me and sometimes with me. I always knew you would do everything in your power to help me. You are one in a million.

So much love for my amazing nieces who, regardless of their age, came running to jump into my arms.

I cannot thank enough my beta readers Tiara Inserto, Katy Durant, Ellen Kirschman, Sharlene Neal, Jolene Soliman, Alex Swanner, Jennifer Wineman, and Les Freeman who weren't just beta readers but powerful voices of encouragement.

To Brooke Warner, the second person to hug my manuscript. I walked aimlessly around the edges of the literary world looking for a way in and a safe place to turn my chicken scratch into a real book. Brooke Warner's dreams are to make other people's dreams come true. So, I thank you, Brooke for your time and guidance to make my dream come true. I also owe a big thank you to editors extraordinaire, Krissa Lagos and Lorraine White.

And to every single person who loved me unconditionally as I trudged through my hell. I would not be here without all of you.

ABOUT THE AUTHOR

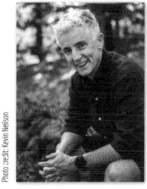

Christy Warren is a retired fire captain from the Berkeley Fire Department. She has twenty-five years of service as a professional paramedic, with seventeen years as a professional firefighter. She was diagnosed with PTSD in 2014 and spent several years recovering. Since retiring from the fire service, she competes in triathlons, has completed the Escape from Alcatraz swim five times, and obtained a bachelor's degree in business from Washington State University. She is a volunteer at the West Coast Post Trauma Retreat and the host of *The Firefighter Deconstructed* podcast. She lives in Pleasant Hill, California, with her wife, Lisa, and her dog, Harriet.

SELECTED TITLES FROM SHE WRITES PRESS

She Writes Press is an independent publishing company
founded to serve women writers everywhere.
Visit us at www.shewritespress.com.

Accidental Soldier: A Memoir of Service and Sacrifice in the Israel Defense Forces by Dorit Sasson. $17.95, 978-1-63152-035-8. When nineteen-year-old Dorit Sasson realized she had no choice but to distance herself from her neurotic, worrywart of a mother in order to become her own person, she volunteered for the Israel Defense Forces—and found her path to freedom.

Army Wife: A Story of Love and Family in the Heart of the Army by Vicki Cody. $16.95, 978-1-63152-127-0. A rare glimpse into the heart of the Army, as seen through the eyes of Vicki Cody, an Army wife of thirty-three years who fell in love with a lieutenant and stayed by his side as he rose up through the ranks, all the way to four-star general and Vice Chief of Staff of the Army.

Headstrong: Surviving a Traumatic Brain Injury by JoAnne Silver Jones. $16.95, 978-1-63152-612-1. After a sudden assault by a stranger left JoAnne Jones with severe traumatic brain injury (TBI), fractured hands, and PTSD, she learned—with the help of a community that gave her the foundations of hope—to live with TBI in a society bursting with violence.

Searching for Normal: The Story of a Girl Gone Too Soon by Karen Meadows. $16.95, 978-1-63152-137-9. Karen Meadows intertwines her own story with excerpts from her daughter Sadie's journals to describes their roller coaster ride through Sadie's depression and a maze of inadequate mental health treatment and services—one that ended with Sadie's suicide at age eighteen.

The Art of Losing it: A Memoir of Grief and Addiction by Rosemary Keevil. $16.95, 978-1-63152-777-7. When her husband dies of cancer and her brother dies of AIDS in the same year, Rosemary is left to raise her two young daughters on her own and plunged into a hurricane of grief—a hurricane from which she seeks refuge in drugs and alcohol.

All the Ghosts Dance Free: A Memoir by Terry Cameron Baldwin. $16.95, 978-1-63152-822-4. A poetic memoir that explores the legacy of alcoholism and teen suicide in one woman's life—and her efforts to create an authentic existence in the face of that legacy.